Intensive Care Unit Telemedicine

Editor

KIANOUSH B. KASHANI

CRITICAL CARE CLINICS

www.criticalcare.theclinics.com

Consulting Editor
JOHN A. KELLUM

July 2019 • Volume 35 • Number 3

ELSEVIER

1600 John F. Kennedy Boulevard • Suite 1800 • Philadelphia, Pennsylvania, 19103-2899

http://www.theclinics.com

CRITICAL CARE CLINICS Volume 35, Number 3
July 2019 ISSN 0749-0704, ISBN-13: 978-0-323-68214-5

Editor: Colleen Dietzler
Developmental Editor: Casey Potter

Critical Care Clinics (ISSN: 0749-0704) is published quarterly by Elsevier Inc., 360 Park Avenue South, New York, NY 10010-1710. Months of issue are January, April, July, and October. Business and Editorial Offices: 1600 John F. Kennedy Blvd., Suite 1800, Philadelphia, PA 19103-2899. Customer Service Office: 6277 Sea Harbor Drive, Orlando, FL 32887-4800. Periodicals postage paid at New York, NY and additional mailing offices. Subscription prices are $243.00 per year for US individuals, $650.00 per year for US institution, $100.00 per year for US students and residents, $285.00 per year for Canadian individuals, $815.00 per year for Canadian institutions, $315.00 per year for international individuals, $815.00 per year for international institutions and $150.00 per year for Canadian and foreign students/residents. To receive student/resident rate, orders must be accompanied by name of affiliated institution, date of term, and the signature of program/residency coordinator on institution letterhead. Orders will be billed at individual rate until proof of status is received. Foreign air speed delivery is included in all *Clinics* subscription prices. All prices are subject to change without notice. POSTMASTER: Send address changes to *Critical Care Clinics*, Elsevier Periodicals Customer Service, 11830 Westline Industrial Drive, St. Louis, MO 63146. **Customer Service: 1-800-654-2452 (US). From outside of the US, call 1-314-447-8871. Fax: 1-314-447-8029. E-mail: journalscustomerservice-usa@ elsevier.com (for print support) or journalsonlinesupport-usa@elsevier.com (for online support).**

Reprints. For copies of 100 or more of articles in this publication, please contact the Commercial Reprints Department, Elsevier Inc., 360 Park Avenue South, New York, NY 10010-1710. Tel.: 212-633-3874; Fax: 212-633-3820; E-mail: reprints@elsevier.com.

Critical Care Clinics is also published in Spanish by Editorial Inter-Medica, Junin 917, 1er A, 1113, Buenos Aires, Argentina.

Critical Care Clinics is covered in *MEDLINE/PubMed (Index Medicus), EMBASE/Excerpta Medica, Current Concepts/ Clinical Medicine, ISI/BIOMED,* and *Chemical Abstracts.*

Contributors

CONSULTING EDITOR

JOHN A. KELLUM, MD, MCCM
Professor, Critical Care Medicine, Medicine, Bioengineering and Clinical and Translational Science, Director, Center for Critical Care Nephrology, Vice Chair for Research, Department of Critical Care Medicine, University of Pittsburgh School of Medicine, Pittsburgh, Pennsylvania, USA

EDITOR

KIANOUSH B. KASHANI, MD, MS
Divisions of Nephrology and Hypertension, and Pulmonary and Critical Care Medicine, Department of Medicine, Mayo Clinic, Rochester, Minnesota, USA

AUTHORS

OMAR BADAWI, PharmD, MPH, FCCM
Research Affiliate, Laboratory for Computational Physiology, Massachusetts Institute of Technology, Cambridge, Massachusetts, USA; Director of Clinical Analytics and Reporting, Patient Care Analytics, Philips Healthcare, Department of Pharmacy Practice and Science, Adjunct Assistant Professor, University of Maryland School of Pharmacy, Baltimore, Maryland, USA

WILLIAM BENDER, MD, MPH
Assistant Professor of Medicine, Division of Pulmonary, Allergy, Critical Care and Sleep Medicine, Emory University School of Medicine, Atlanta, Georgia, USA

IRIS BERMAN, MSN, BSN, RN, CCRN-K
VP, Telehealth Services, Northwell Health, Syosset, New York, USA

TOM BOBICH, MBA
VP, Marketing, Advanced ICU Care, Irvine, California, USA

THERESA BRINDISE, MS, BSN, RN
AdvocateAuroraHealth, Director, eICU, Oak Brook, Illinois, USA

TIMOTHY G. BUCHMAN, PhD, MD, FACS, FCCP, MCCM
Professor of Surgery, Anesthesiology, and Biomedical Informatics, Emory University School of Medicine, Atlanta, Georgia, USA

SEAN M. CAPLES, DO, MS
Medical Director, The Enhanced Critical Care Program, Division of Pulmonary and Critical Care Medicine, Mayo Clinic, Rochester, Minnesota, USA

LEO ANTHONY CELI, MD, MS, MPH
Clinical Research Director, Principal Research Scientist, Laboratory for Computational Physiology, Massachusetts Institute of Technology, Cambridge, Massachusetts, USA;

Staff Physician, Department of Pulmonary, Critical Care, and Sleep Medicine, Beth Israel Deaconess Medical Center, Boston, Massachusetts, USA

THERESA DAVIS, PhD, RN, NE-BC, FAAN
Clinical Operations Director, enVision eICU Inova Telemedicine, Falls Church, Virginia, USA

JOSEPH CHRISTOPHER FARMER, MD, FACP, FCCP, FCCM
Emeritus Professor and Chair, Mayo Clinic, Rochester, Minnesota, USA; Clinical Consultant and eIntensivist, Avera eCare, Avera Healthcare, Sioux Falls, South Dakota, USA; Senior Critical Care Consultant and Healthcare System Advisor, VinMec Healthcare System, Hà Nội, Vietnam

PRAMOD K. GURU, MBBS, MD
Department of Critical Care Medicine, Mayo Clinic, Jacksonville, Florida, USA

VITALY HERASEVICH, MD, PhD, FCCM
Professor of Anesthesiology and Medicine, Department of Anesthesiology and Perioperative Medicine, Division of Critical Care, Mayo Clinic, Rochester, Minnesota, USA

CHERYL A. HIDDLESON, MSN, RN, CENP, CCRN-E
Director, Emory eICU Center, Emory Healthcare Inc., Atlanta, Georgia, USA

ANNIE B. JOHNSON, MSN, CNP
Instructor of Surgery, Critical Care Nurse Practitioner, Department of Pulmonary and Critical Care Medicine, Mayo Clinic, Rochester, Minnesota, USA

SANDRA L. KANE-GILL, PharmD, MSc, FCCM, FCCP
Professor of Pharmacy, Critical Care Medicine, Biomedical Informatics and Clinical Translational Science Institute, University of Pittsburgh, Pittsburgh, Pennsylvania, USA

RYAN D. KINDLE, MD
Research Affiliate, Laboratory for Computational Physiology, Massachusetts Institute of Technology, Cambridge, Massachusetts, USA; Clinical Research Fellow, Department of Pulmonary, Critical Care, and Sleep Medicine, Beth Israel Deaconess Medical Center, Boston, Massachusetts, USA

ISABELLE C. KOPEC, MD, FACP, FCCP
Vice President of Medical Affairs and Co-Founder, Advanced ICU Care, St Louis, Missouri, USA; Chair, Department of Critical Care Medicine, SSM DePaul, Bridgeton, Missouri, USA

CRAIG M. LILLY, MD
Professor, Departments of Medicine, Anesthesiology, and Surgery, Clinical and Population Health Research Program, University of Massachusetts Medical School, Graduate School of Biomedical Sciences, UMass Memorial Health Care, Memorial Medical Center, Worcester, Massachusetts, USA

JARED T. MICKELSON, DO
Fellow, Division of Pulmonary and Critical Care, Department of Medicine, University of Massachusetts Medical School, Graduate School of Biomedical Sciences, UMass Memorial Health Care, Memorial Medical Center, Worcester, Massachusetts, USA

PABLO MORENO FRANCO, MD
Division of Transplant Medicine, Department of Critical Care Medicine, Mayo Clinic, Jacksonville, Florida, USA

FRED RINCON, MD, MSc, MBE, FACP, FCCP, FCCM
Associate Professor of Neurology and Neurological Surgery, Department of Neurosurgery, Thomas Jefferson University, Philadelphia, Pennsylvania, USA

TERESA RINCON, PhD, RN, CCRN-K, FCCM
Director of Clinical Operations/Innovation, TeleHealth, UMassMemorial Health Care, Worcester, Massachusetts, USA

DEVANG K. SANGHAVI, MBBS, MD
Department of Critical Care Medicine, Mayo Clinic, Jacksonville, Florida, USA

SHAWN STURLAND, MBChB, FANZCA, FCICM
Visiting Research Scientist, Laboratory for Computational Physiology, Massachusetts Institute of Technology, Cambridge, Massachusetts, USA; Clinical Executive Director of Quality Improvement and Patient Safety, Department of Intensive Care, Wellington Hospital, Wellington, New Zealand

SANJAY SUBRAMANIAN, MD, MMM
Associate Professor, Department of Anesthesiology, Division of Critical Care, Washington University in St. Louis, St Louis, Missouri, USA

CINDY WELSH, RN, MBA, FACHE
VP, Adult Critical Care, eICU, Advocate Intensivist Partners, AdvocateAuroraHealth, Oak Brook, Illinois, USA

Contents

Conceptualizing, designing, implementing, and sustaining a successful critical care telemedicine program is a complex undertaking. All of these steps must be fully accomplished as a joint effort between a host facility and the telemedicine service provider. Important administrative considerations that must be incorporated into planning and execution steps include managing change. We briefly discuss critical aspects of establishing a sustainable business model, and aligning the critical care telemedicine program with institutional vision, goals, and mission. Discussed are important telemedicine provider infrastructure, key personnel considerations, and how a program defines and measures value.

Telehealth in intensive care units (TeleICU) is the provision of critical care using audio-visual communication and health information systems across varying clinical and geographically dispersed settings. The optimal structure of a TeleICU team is one that leverages expert clinical knowledge to address the needs of critical care patients, regardless of hospital location or availability of an onsite intensivist. Information related to the optimal TeleICU team structure is lacking. This article examines the optimal TeleICU team composition, which is one that incorporates the use of an interdisciplinary approach, leverages technology, and is cognizant of varying geographic locations.

Tele-ICU improves access to high-quality critical care using a variety of information technology (IT) solutions. Recent advances in computing and telecommunications have expanded telemedicine programs nationwide. This review covers the basic principles of delivery models, technological needs, cybersecurity, health IT standards, and interoperability required for a Tele-ICU system. This will enable a better definition of Tele-ICU platforms and build robust programs.

Intensive care unit (ICU) telemedicine lowers mortality, shortens length of stay and improves best practice compliance when implemented effectively. As a review of the literature shows, program success is not guaranteed. The model of ICU telemedicine with published results is the one designed to leverage an intensivist-led remote critical care team, assisted by technology, data streaming, and analytics. The value of ICU telemedicine lies in how well the model is applied, leveraged, and integrated into the existing staff, structure, and processes at the bedside. Key domains to master to achieve this integration are discussed.

The health care delivery system is complex. New technologies offer new treatment options. The process of quality improvement includes system re-engineering. Telemedicine intensive care is an evolving area of delivery. Its core characteristic is the need for a merger of human and machine activity. Optimal use of quality improvement tools can lead to improved patient-centered outcomes. This article outlines how quality improvement tools can be used to facilitate the patient-centered collaboration with a focus on defining evidence-practice gaps, developing actionable metrics, analyzing the impact of proposed interventions, quantifying resources, prioritizing improvement plans, evaluating results, and diffusing best practices.

Advances in clinical information sciences, telecommunication technologies, electronic health records, early warning systems, automated acuity assessment, and clinician communication support systems have allowed current-generation intensive care (ICU) telemedicine systems to address the inefficiencies of the failed advice-upon-request ICU telemedicine model. Value is related to the ability of health care systems to leverage ICU telemedicine resources to provide care. Local financial benefits of ICU telemedicine program implementation depend on changing behavior to better focus on activities that reduce the duration of critical illness and length of stay.

This review outlines various care models used in tele–intensive care unit (tele-ICU) programs. They may be differentiated by personnel and approach to care. Low-intensity models, such as nocturnal coverage, may be adequate for some ICU practices. Others might benefit from a high-intensity model, especially those practices that desire a proactive approach to care. Also discussed is the incorporation of the education of trainees into tele-ICU models.

This article examines the history of the telemedicine intensive care unit (tele-ICU), the current state of clinical decision support systems (CDSS) in the tele-ICU, applications of machine learning (ML) algorithms to critical care, and opportunities to integrate ML with tele-ICU CDSS. The enormous quantities of data generated by tele-ICU systems is a major driver in the development of the large, comprehensive, heterogeneous, and granular data sets necessary to develop generalizable ML CDSS algorithms, and deidentification of these data sets expands opportunities for ML CDSS research.

Intensive care unit (ICU) telemedicine is an established entity that has the ability to not only improve the effectiveness, efficiency, and safety of critical care, but to also serve as a tool to combat staffing shortages and resource-limited environments. Several areas for future innovation exist within the field, including the use of advanced practice providers, robust inclusion in medical education, and concurrent application of advanced machine learning. The globalization of critical care services will also likely be predominantly delivered by ICU telemedicine. Limitations faced by the field include technical issues, financial concerns, and organizational elements.

For well over a decade, intensive care unit (ICU) telemedicine programs have been providing care to patients and families and an invaluable service to many receiving sites that are otherwise outside the traditional reach of high-quality critical care. It will be important that during this growth, outcomes regarding the unique services provided by ICU telemedicine are accurately measured, not the least of which is nursing, provider, and patient and family satisfaction. More work is required to ensure that the voices of those most intimately affected by ICU telemedicine services are heard and that programs are evaluated and adapted in response to these outcomes.

As more specialized care gets centralized in centers of excellence, patients admitted to rural hospitals may be at a disadvantage at the time of accessing expertise or receiving advanced care. In this setting, telemedicine models provide a justification to equalize care across different levels. The diversity in telemedicine services is vast and is expanding. Even with all the subsets of telemedicine, including telepharmacy, telestroke, teledialysis, and tele–emergency medicine, the reasons for providing services and associated limitations are similar. However, there is a lack of empirical research including best practices and resultant outcomes for these subsets of telemedicine models.

CRITICAL CARE CLINICS

SERIES OF RELATED INTEREST

Emergency Medicine Clinics
Available at: https://www.emed.theclinics.com/

THE CLINICS ARE AVAILABLE ONLINE!
Access your subscription at:
www.theclinics.com

Preface

Telemedicine in Intensive Care Units: A Luxury or Necessity?

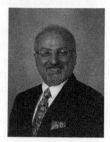

Kianoush B. Kashani, MD, MS
Editor

The advent of telemedicine programs and their utilization in intensive care units (ICU), started in the 1970s, was initially designed to enhance the ability of local providers by simple verbal or video consultation with an ICU expert. Over the course of years with evolution of clinical informatics and connectivity, the idea has grown to the contemporary Tele-ICU practices, which not only provide expert opinion to the local providers but also offer a wide range of services, including monitoring, supervisions, communications with patients, families, and local providers of many disciplines, active resuscitation and stabilization, optimization, and deescalation processes for critically ill patients in shock, and additional services, including Tele-pharmacy, Tele-dialysis, Tele-stroke, and so forth.

Over the course of the past four decades, one can witness the progressive use of more modern and advanced technological tools to provide appropriate care to the patients at need. This not only includes better communication tools and video-connectivity devices but also the use of more advanced artificial intelligence and clinical decision support systems, which has provided a tremendous opportunity to provide safer and more efficient and timely care. While some use Tele-ICU services to enhance the safety of their own local ICU practices, the majority of organizations offer such services to the remote ICUs that have limited availabilities of experts throughout the day and week. This has opened a whole new horizon for the ability of clinicians to provide high-quality critical care in underserved areas throughout the globe.

Building an infrastructure of Tele-ICU and maintaining it are not minuscule tasks, and barriers like legal hurdles, need for accreditation, and appropriate training and licensing could limit the spectrum of what could be done using Tele-ICU. Having said that, the growth of several active and effective Tele-ICU programs has paved the way for other institutions to offer or receive such services. One crucial

Crit Care Clin 35 (2019) xi–xii
https://doi.org/10.1016/j.ccc.2019.03.001
0749-0704/19/© 2019 Published by Elsevier Inc.

administrative aspect of Tele-ICU is constant monitoring for cost-effectiveness of services to enhance the viability of these programs.

One of the essential aspects of Tele-ICU is the need for growing knowledge regarding the best practices to improve outcomes and provider, receiver, patient, and family satisfaction. Therefore, focusing on Tele-ICU–centered research and quality improvement projects is essential in providing ever-improving care to the most vulnerable patients in ICUs. Innovative projects to employ new technologies for care enhancement are an absolutely necessary to allow the practice of Tele-ICU to grow beyond the current level of sophistication.

The other important factor to be considered is the multidisciplinary nature of Tele-ICU care. The successful Tele-ICU provider programs (Hub) are those that have been able to make and maintain teams of nurses, pharmacists, advanced clinical practitioners, respiratory therapists, information technologists, secretaries, and intensive care and other subspecialty physicians that provide services to multiple disciplines in the receiving (Spoke) ICUs. Without appropriate organization and communication, often the care would not be optimized, which increases the chances of harm and missed opportunities and increases cost.

Critical Care Clinics recognizes the importance of this new path for providing appropriate care to ICU patients and hence has dedicated this issue to the topic of Tele-ICU. In this issue of *Critical Care Clinics*, several world experts in the field share their vast knowledge and experience regarding different aspects of Tele-ICU programs. We start with the administrative and legal requirements for initiation and maintenance of a Tele-ICU program, including accreditation processes. Then, we focus on the current state and future of technological aspects of successful Tele-ICU programs before concentrating on the organization of optimum teams and models of care that could be offered by Tele-ICU. We then report the impact of Tele-ICU on critically ill patient outcomes, how to maintain the quality of care, patient/provider satisfaction, and cost-effectiveness of Tele-ICU programs. We also describe some of the recently described innovations and recognized limitations of these programs along with a variety of services that could be provided using the Tele-ICU infrastructure. This issue offers a wide range of ideas for future practice improvements and research projects, which it is hoped translates to improved outcomes of ICU patients' recipient of these services.

Kianoush B. Kashani, MD, MS
Division of Nephrology and Hypertension
Division of Pulmonary and
Critical Care Medicine
Department of Medicine
Mayo Clinic
200 First Street Southwest
Rochester, MN 55905, USA

E-mail address:
kashani.kianoush@mayo.edu

Important Administrative Aspects of Critical Care Telemedicine Programs

Joseph Christopher Farmer, MD, FCCP, FCCM[a,b,c,*]

KEYWORDS

- Telemedicine • Critical care • Organizational structure • Financial models
- Personnel management • Balanced scorecard • Quality metrics

KEY POINTS

- Before implementing any telemedicine activity, it is important to fully define *all* nonclinical requirements of the program.
- A key success metric of any telemedicine program is sustainability.
- Important nonclinical program requirements include the following:
  - Fiscal viability.
  - Robust information technology and networking infrastructure.
  - Comprehensive licensing and credentialing capabilities.
  - Robust training programs.
  - Quality programs infrastructure.
  - Demonstrating value.

INTRODUCTION

Early generations telemedicine were commonly built on a foundation of evangelism and hope. The "shiny objects" aspect of this new technology convinced many that telemedicine was an ingenious solution for a wide range of difficult care situations.[1] It was and still is ingenious, but was commonly implemented quickly and with limited support structures in place. This was a common lapse; forgetting that technology is a tool, not a solution. And unfortunately, when new technology is not embraced by

Disclosure Statement: The Trajectory Group, LLC, owner and president. The author serves as a health care management consultant and provides remunerated consulting services for Avera eCare and VinMec Healthcare including the domains of telemedicine and connected eCare.
[a] Mayo Clinic, Rochester, MN, USA; [b] Avera eCare, Avera Healthcare, Sioux Falls, SD, USA; [c] VinMec Healthcare System, Hà Nội, Viet Nam
* Mayo Clinic Emeriti Association and Faculty Office, Mayo Clinic in Arizona, 13400 East Shea Boulevard, Scottsdale, AZ 85259.
E-mail address: farmer.j@mayo.edu

Crit Care Clin 35 (2019) 407–414
https://doi.org/10.1016/j.ccc.2019.02.001
0749-0704/19/© 2019 Elsevier Inc. All rights reserved.
criticalcare.theclinics.com

"nonevangelists," it is usually not sustainable and often does not succeed. Numerous early telemedicine programs were initiated with the hope that value would simply happen. But, as we know, "hope is not a strategy."

The equipment of many earlier telemedicine programs was eventually consigned to storage closets. This further reinforced the negative perspective held by many regarding the day-to-day value of telemedicine. The memories of these earlier failed initiatives continue to deter successful implementation of some telemedicine programs today.[2]

The successful development, implementation, and adoption of telemedicine programs should begin with these questions[3]:

- Is there an actual *demand* for the telemedicine program? Remember, "need," and "demand" are not the same thing (see later in this article). Adoption is ultimately about change management, and people will not change how they do things unless they endorse an imperative for change.[4]
- For the host facility, health care professionals, does the proposed telemedicine activity lessen *my* workload, improve *my* efficiency, and enhance the care of *my* patients?
- For host facility health care professionals, am I fully confident in the clinical abilities of the telemedicine staff who will provide clinical surveillance and interventions for my patients?
- For the host facility leaders, is the cost of the proposed telemedicine program reasonable and sustainable?
- For the telemedicine services provider, is the responsibility and "burden" of providing telemedicine sustainable? Total system costs versus revenue stream? What about information technology infrastructure requirements like accessing multiple electronic health records or other existing clinical systems at a host facility?
- Consider telemedicine staff recruitment? Staff training requirements? Physician credentialing? Staff satisfaction? For telemedicine professionals, they ask, "will I make a difference, will I be valued and treated with mutual respect, will the technology burden be acceptable to me?"
- Does the proposed telemedicine service demonstrate tangible value for a host facility? Patient safety? Quality? Efficiency gains?

DISCUSSION

In this section, we review several essentials regarding the development and implementation of a successful critical care telemedicine program.[5,6] Given our space constraints, this is not comprehensive. Therefore, I will enumerate and review these selective program considerations concisely, but not in their entirety. Some of this discussion reflects the published experiences of others, but some of this also reflects my personal opinions, based on my career experiences with programmatic development. **Table 1** offers a checklist of some of the major challenges that should be considered when developing a critical care telemedicine program.

Change Management: Capturing the Demand Versus Identifying the Need

This could also be called "winning hearts and minds." A fundamental difference between "need" and "demand" is desire. Oftentimes, "need" is first recognized by institutional leaders, administrators, and others. They recognize internal care processes inefficiency (eg, length of stay, lack of beds), potential quality lapses, confusing clinical

Table 1
Important development considerations for critical care telemedicine

Domain	Relevant Considerations
Plans, goals, and mission alignment	• What exactly and precisely are you trying to accomplish with an intensive care unit (ICU) telemedicine system? • Did you conduct a comprehensive institutional assessment, as well as a market analysis of the host facility/s or community/s? • Which clinical services lines have anticipated growth, and what are their critical care needs? • What are the current local ICU physician capabilities, and will they satisfy these anticipated demands?
Change management	Differentiate "need" vs "demand." • Is there an acknowledged imperative for this change? • Will ICU telemedicine improve workflow, care quality, efficiency, and overall performance of the involved ICUs? • Are these planned improvements measurable? • Do a majority of the host facility intensivists support these changes? If "no," is their lack of support modifiable? • Does the planning process include intensivists and other hospital-based physicians from the host facility/s?
Business model	• Does your business model require grants funding/ foundation endowments/institutional stipends? • If "yes," where will this be obtained and will it be necessary beyond a start-up phase? • Have you completed a comprehensive cost evaluation of all aspects of the telemedicine program? This includes not only the equipment and telemedicine maintenance costs, but also all administrative personnel, physician salary support, licensing and credentialing, physical plant(s), training costs, marketing, sales, and so forth. • How will you model revenue cost savings? Quality, workflow efficiency, throughput gains, patient complication avoidance, and so forth.
Infrastructure	Do you have the following infrastructure in place? • Staff training (host facility and telemedicine provider) • Telemedicine staff scheduling and other administrative support • Medical staff professionals licensing and credentialing (oftentimes multi-state) • Clinical protocols • Maintenance of training • Billing and account management, human resources, and salary support • Quality review programs • Operational protocols • Health Insurance Portability and Accountability Act and privacy surveillance
Critical care telemedicine physicians	• What is the selected personnel staffing model for critical care telemedicine physicians? Full-time employment, part-time employment, other? • If you choose the latter, will you provide benefits to part-time workers? • How will you infuse institutional culture, loyalty, performance goals, and accountability into the daily activities of critical care telemedicine physicians?

(continued on next page)

Table 1 (continued)	
Domain	**Relevant Considerations**
Value measurement	• How will you define and measure quality? • How will these quality metrics be measured quantified? • Will you assess impact? If "yes," what does that mean and how will you credibly measure and quantify impact? • Did you actively involve host facility finance leaders in the development of the business model that translates quality improvement, adverse events avoidance, and facility efficiency gains into imputed cost savings? • How will you reliably calculate "value?"

coverage models, nursing distress with delayed physician decision making or difficulty accessing clinicians, and others. They seek to more reliably fill these gaps.

In a classic "us versus them" mindset, these individuals are sometimes described by physicians as, "administrators who won't actually use the telemedicine system themselves." Then, "administrators" ask, "what can we do to rectify these problems?" And so, a problem begins: the *initiators* are viewed negatively, and the *effectors* who will interface with the telemedicine system are placed into a defensive posture from the outset of "problem-solving" discussions.

Instead, recognize this as an opportunity to help well-intentioned clinicians (who work very hard) make their lives better. Understand that a root cause for many of these issues is that they are "stretched too thin." Exasperation ensues. We should begin by allowing these clinicians to discuss their needs. This is not just telemedicine. First, understand their day-to-day concerns. Make lists. Discuss ways to help them accomplish their tasks more effectively. Then align these with the needs of institutional leaders; enumerate commonality. This translates "need" into "demand." Life is negotiation, so is telemedicine.

Building a Sustainable Business Model

When you review business models of existing telemedicine programs, several common themes emerge. First, many telemedicine programs successfully obtain grant funding that defrays some costs: initial funding for rooms or buildings, outfitting hubs, initial staffing, ongoing infrastructure costs, quality infrastructure, and so on. Some of this money comes from traditional research funding sources, but some funds are provided by philanthropic foundations or institutional endowments. This impacts longer-term finances; unless the business model evolves, finding follow-on grants and stipends become imperative for ongoing sustainability.

Next, understand that a 24/7 intensive care unit (ICU) telemedicine surveillance model is very expensive. Consider the following from a 2009 publication by Berenson colleagues[7]:

Cost was the major consideration affecting adoption. For eICU implementation, according to VISICU, discounted costs range from about $30,000 to $50,000 per ICU bed. Therefore, the cost of equipping 100 ICU beds is approximately $3–$5 million. VISICU's estimates of annual operating costs were approximately 20% of the software costs or about $300,000 for 100 beds. Staffing costs depend on hours in use and level of additional staff in the off-site center; typical staffing scenarios add approximately $1–$2 million per year per 100 beds covered. Adding to the cost considerations, virtually no third-party payers pay for the professional services of the physicians and nurses staffing the eICU control center.

This also does not include the eICU equipment costs to the telemedicine provider. It also does not include staffing and other infrastructure costs of the telemedicine provider. Who can reasonably afford all of this in today's dollars? Given that these services are not typically reimbursable, program fee structure is by subscription. Therefore, getting to a mutually sustainable return on investment (ROI) for service providers *and* host institutions becomes very challenging when a significant proportion of the total monetary stream goes to a third-party vendor. Moreover, as we discuss in the staffing section, this directly impacts *how* eICU programs employ physician staff. For our future, I do not think that this is a sustainable business model.

ROI is commonly modeled using "soft money," cost avoidance estimates rather than measuring direct dollars saved. What are the authentic costs savings of improved care quality and inpatient throughput (efficiency gains)? These numbers vary widely according to the financial modeling approach that is deployed. When compared with hard number costs of the telemedicine system, imputing soft number institutional savings creates skepticism. Ultimately, this complicates efforts to quantify "value."

Finally, one must ask, is a 24/7 ICU telemedicine surveillance model really required? Does presumed benefit truly justify its high cost? Or, can the ICU surveillance model be variably designed by each institution? Daily ICU rounds combined with acute event response capabilities may be sufficient for many. I think that the solution approach can vary according to specific institutional needs: we don't all wear the same size or style shoes? Aggregate ICU acuity of illness, types of ICU patients served, on-site ICU clinician care model, and ICU telemedicine programmatic goals should all be considered as well. Cost and need should be well aligned with the ICU model of telemedicine care. There is not a single approach that reliably ensures this alignment because the needs and structures of each program vary widely; this must be individually determined.

Aligning "the Plan" with Host Facility Goals and Mission

What exactly and precisely are you trying to accomplish with an ICU telemedicine system? This means that a prospective ICU telemedicine site should first conduct a comprehensive institutional assessment, as well as a market analysis of their community. How does this align with the institution's mission and goals? What are the current and future medical needs of the community that may impact critical care? Which clinical services lines have anticipated growth, and what are their critical care needs? What are the current local ICU physician capabilities, and will they satisfy these anticipated demands? Are community physicians interested in participating in a telemedicine service model?

The answers to these questions should be well aligned with your proposed telemedicine service model. All of this should be clearly defined and enumerated *before* building the ICU telemedicine program. Failure to do this can result in rejection or nonacceptance of "that program" by "the locals." Furthermore, I view the role of an ICU telemedicine group as an active partner in these institutional planning processes, and not merely the eventual service provider.

Necessary Telemedicine Provider Infrastructure

The technology is the (relatively) easy part. As we have already discussed, funding can be an enormous challenge. In addition, there is staff training (host facility and telemedicine provider), telemedicine staff scheduling, and other administrative support, medical staff professionals licensing and credentialing (oftentimes multi-state), clinical protocols development, maintenance of training, billing and account management, human resources and salary support, quality review programs development, operational protocols development, Health Insurance Portability and Accountability Act and privacy surveillance, and finally, even more training. This is a substantial cost burden to be absorbed by a telemedicine service provider.

Before an ICU telemedicine program can launch, you must decide exactly what you will do and how you will do it. This means clinical and operational protocols development. Some of this is similar to Rapid Response Teams program protocols, including things like Situation-Background-Assessment-Recommendation communication tools. Other communications protocols need to be formally defined as well. Workflow integration also benefits from defined choreography. That is, how does telemedicine fit into the daily routine of a host facility ICU.

Care bundles implementation are also important, for example, how will you diagnose and manage sepsis? Implement A-B-C-D-E-F bundles? What are mutually preferred treatment strategies for common ICU clinical problems? Improved host facility adherence to best clinical practices is a clear goal of an ICU telemedicine system.

Operationally, how will ICU telemedicine clinical staff communicate with host facility physician staff about ICU telemedicine interventions and activities? Emergency response protocols require delineation as well. Structured handover protocols for ICU telemedicine staff should also be in place. Everyone needs to be trained regarding collaboration, how to fit into routines, interfacing with non-ICU professionals like clinical pharmacy, physical therapy/occupational therapy, medical imaging, and others. These are examples; there are many other operational considerations.

Training requirements for everyone are substantial and ongoing. I will not enumerate each of these, but rather highlight other training opportunities that enhance collaboration. Clinical training can be used as a "bridge builder" between ICU telemedicine staff and host facility staff. For example, mutually conducting a Fundamental Critical Care Support course and Advanced Cardiac Life Support course are examples of educational cooperation. Also, consider ICU telemedicine staff teaching and assisting with host facility care bundle implementation, like the A-B-C-D-E-F bundle.

If an ICU telemedicine service provider works with multiple host hospitals, that likely means multiple electronic health records (EHRs). This is a substantial training burden for similar but different physician order entry, as well as myriad other processes. For example, under what circumstances are telemedicine staff expected to write progress or events notes in the EHR? If that physician is following beyond a predefined threshold of eICU patient coverage, this is problematic.

Licensing and credentialing of professional staff can be significantly burdensome, requiring dedicated telemedicine provider credentials staff. Each state and hospital has individual requirements and processes. These requirements are commonly overlapping, and many use outdated manual processes. Checkbox paper forms, faxes, individual notarization, and e-mailed PDFs are still the rule for many. The intent is to ensure the public safety and welfare through close surveillance of physician licensing and credentialing, as well as other clinical staff. Unfortunately and in my opinion, these highly individualized manual approaches by many states and facilities may actually hinder awareness across boundaries regarding competency or other patient care breaches. Ultimately, this results in an extensive administrative burden for licensing and credentialing staff at a telemedicine center.

External accreditation of telemedicine programs as well as defined accreditation standards are not yet widely accepted. During 2018, 2 organizations announced their initiation of voluntary telemedicine accreditation pathways for telemedicine programs.[8,9] These organizations are not critical care specific, and include both inpatient and ambulatory telemedicine accreditation activities. The first is a nonprofit organization in Washington, DC: the Utilization Review Accreditation Commission. They call themselves "the first independent, third-party national program to offer comprehensive oversight of diverse telehealth programs." The second organization is the ClearHealth Quality Institute (CHQI), also in the national capital region. CHQI is partnered with the American Telemedicine Association for their standards definitions.

Selected Personnel Considerations

Most ICU telemedicine physicians are part-time eICU workers. They typically have another "day job." For many centers that means physicians split their time between bedside critical care working in an ICU and telemedicine critical care. Many of these physicians are employed and salaried by an organization or institution that provides both bedside critical care and telemedicine critical care. Telemedicine in one component of their activities that constitute their total salary. They may receive an additional stipend for their telemedicine efforts. Most of these physicians also receive benefits along with their salary. In another model, critical care physicians are recruited by a telemedicine program to work part-time and "cover shifts." These individuals are remunerated either by an annual amount, an hourly payment rate, or by the shift. As "part-timers," they often do not receive benefits from the institution or organization for this work.

Keys to high-quality medicine include professional staff satisfaction, embracing an institutional culture for excellence, philosophic (clinical) consistency among physicians, peer-to-peer collaboration, excellent communications, setting clear expectations, and accountability. The first practice model described is aligned with these goals. The second model poses some challenges. It would be easy for physicians in this model to view this as "extra income" without a sense of belonging. Telemedicine acceptance by host facility users is fragile; therefore, providing excellent "customer service" is essential. Without a significant effort to define and maintain clear performance expectations, the second model carries a risk of an itinerant "shift worker" mindset.

Defining and Measuring the Value

Value (quality/cost) is variably defined. For most critical care telemedicine programs, calculating direct financial costs is straightforward. However, defining and measuring quality is less clear. For critical care telemedicine, quality is mostly assessed as "impact." Examples include interventions that prevent "badness" and/or improve compliance with best practice clinical standards. Assessment of deleterious events prevention is highly subjective, and measurement of compliance with care bundles and published clinical guidelines can be contentious. A specific example of the latter is antibiotic stewardship and deescalation of antimicrobial therapies. Communications from a remote ICU telemedicine physician with an on-site host facility physician to decrease or stop antibiotics sometimes engenders friction and even control issues regarding the ongoing need for patient treatment. In this example, the value is defined more by the quality of the *interactions* between these individuals, as opposed to actual clinical impact.

It is not possible to estimate the overall value of a telemedicine program without subjective modeling (both cost and quality). For example, how many ventilator-associated events (pneumonia) were prevented by ensuring that all ICU patients had the heads of their beds properly elevated, or that they received appropriate oral care or other bundle elements? What was the imputed financial cost of a pneumonia event that was "prevented?"

Therefore, value modeling should be mutually accomplished including both the telemedicine program *and* the host facility. What are the value (impact) goals and priorities for the program? What are the baseline modeling assumptions? What are the metrics and how will these metrics be measured or estimated? Who will "keep score"? What tools are needed? How will "accountability" be applied to achieve overall performance improvement? And last, did you report or publish what you learned?

SUMMARY

I have offered you a glimpse of the administrative issues that must be addressed if you wish to launch a successful critical care telemedicine program. The single highest priority is superb communications between the telemedicine service provider and the host facility during all program planning phases, during program implementation, and routinely during ongoing program use/activities. Success is equally defined by excellent teamwork as well as vigilant patient surveillance and interventions.

REFERENCES

1. Grigsby J, Sanders JH. Telemedicine: where it is and where it's going. Ann Intern Med 1998;129(2):123–7.
2. Grigsby B, Brega AG, Bennett RE, et al. The slow pace of interactive video telemedicine adoption: the perspective of telemedicine program administrators on physician participation, Telemedicine and e-Health. 13.6 2007. p645+, Available at: http://www.liebertpub.com/publication.aspx?pub_id=54. Accessed December 19, 2019.
3. Critical success factors: how to establish a successful telehealth service, Health and Human Services. Victoria (Australia), ISBN 978-0-9924829-8-5. Available at: http://www.health.vic.gov.au/telehealth. Accessed December 19, 2019.
4. Kotter JP. Leading change. 1R edition. Harvard Business Review Press; 2012. ISBN-10: 9781422186435.
5. Framework for the implementation of a telemedicine service. Washington, DC: Pan American Health Organization (PAHO); 2016. ISBN 978-92-75-11903-7.
6. 10 best practices for implementing telemedicine in hospitals. Becker's HEALTH IT & CIO REPORT; 2012. Available at: https://www.beckershospitalreview.com/healthcare-information-technology/10-best-practices-for-implementing-telemedicine-in-hospitals.html.
7. Berenson RA, Grossman JM, November EA. Does telemonitoring of patients—the eICU—improve intensive care? Health Aff (Millwood) 2009;28(5):w937–47.
8. Available at: https://www.urac.org/programs/telehealth-accreditation. Accessed December 19, 2019.
9. Available at: https://www.chqi.com/programs-and-services/telemedicine/. Accessed December 19, 2019.

TeleICU Interdisciplinary Care Teams

Cindy Welsh, RN, MBA[a],*, Teresa Rincon, PhD, RN, CCRN-K[b,1],
Iris Berman, MSN, BSN, RN, CCRN-K[c], Tom Bobich, MBA[d,2], Theresa Brindise, MS, BSN, RN[e,3],
Theresa Davis, PhD, RN, NE-BC[f]

KEYWORDS

- Interdisciplinary • TeleICU • Staffing • Work flow • Remote ICU • TeleICU team
- Intensive care

KEY POINTS

- The composition of the TeleICU team requires several key factors to be evaluated; one size does not fit all.
- Workflows in the TeleICU are established by key stakeholders, including the bedside caregivers and the TeleICU team, while incorporating evidence-based best practices.
- TeleICU technology facilitates collaborative and integrated workflows.

INTRODUCTION

The terms telemedicine and telehealth are considered interchangeable terms by the American Telemedicine Association and are defined as the use of remote health care technologies to deliver health care services.[1] Telehealth in intensive care units (TeleICU) is the provision of critical care using audio-visual communication and health information systems to leverage expertise and decision support systems across varying clinical and geographically dispersed settings.[2,3] TeleICU care includes 2 geographic components: the TeleICU care center (referred to as the "hub" or distant

C. Welsh, I. Berman, T. Bobich, and T. Brindise have no commercial or financial conflicts to disclose. T. Rincon has received travel support (no honorarium) by Philips Healthcare for advisory and speaking roles. T. Davis is a Director on the AACN Board of Directors.
^a Adult Critical Care, eICU, AdvocateAuroraHealth, 1400 Kensington Road, Oak Brook, IL 60523, USA; ^b TeleHealth, UMassMemorial Health Care, 100 Front Street 1st floor, 114H, Worcester, MA 01608, USA; ^c Telehealth Services, Northwell Health, 15 Burke Lane, Syosset, NY 11791, USA; ^d Marketing, Advanced ICU Care, 2040 Main Street Suite 240, Irvine, CA 92614, USA; ^e AdvocateAuroraHealth, eICU, 1400 Kensington Road, Oak Brook, IL 60523, USA; ^f enVision eICU Inova Telemedicine, 8110 Gatehouse Road Suite 600 West, Falls Church, VA 22042, USA
¹ Present address: 100 Front Street, 1st, floor, 114H Worcester, MA 01608.
² Present address: 2040 Main Street, Suite 240, Irvine, CA 92614.
³ Present address: 1400 Kensington Road, Oak Brook, IL 60523.
* Corresponding author. 1400 Kensington Road, Oak Brook, IL 60523.
E-mail address: Cindy.Welsh@advocatehealth.com

site) and the hospital critical care environment (referred to as the origin or spoke site) where the patient is receiving care from the hub with the support of the telemedicine technology.[1,4] This article focuses on the predominant TeleICU model, which uses continuous monitoring and a centralized hub (or multiple hubs). Some TeleICU models use an episodic consultative approach to intervention, whereby distant clinicians intervene remotely only when contacted by the site. The efficacy and cost of this model could be evaluated when considering the use of remote TeleICU.[5–8]

The technology platforms for telehealth include components of hardware, software, and mobile applications (apps) to optimize the surveillance and care of patients for the provider and receiver of services.[3] Information related to the optimal TeleICU team structure is lacking in the literature. This article examines the optimal TeleICU team composition, which is one that incorporates the use of an interdisciplinary approach, leverages technology, and is cognizant of varying geographic locations. In addition, the American Association of Critical Care Nurses (AACN) Synergy Model and Healthy Work Environments (HWE) standards, and the Relational Coordination theoretic foundation, are discussed. Use of these models is important to the development, composition, and success of the TeleICU team.[2,9] Finally, future possibilities for TeleICU team structures and functions are discussed as telemedicine continues to evolve and finds its way into mainstream medicine as an integral component of the health care system.

THE ESSENTIAL TeleICU TEAM STRUCTURE

The optimal structure of a TeleICU team is one that leverages expert clinical knowledge to address the needs of critical care patients, regardless of hospital geography or availability of an onsite intensivist. Early applications in 1999 focused on an intensivist-driven care model working in synergy with expert critical care nurses in the distant site.[10,11] Through the evolution of critical care, the importance of a team approach that combines the efforts of all team members, regardless of their physical location and inclusive of both origin and distant site locations, to achieve optimal care delivery in complex critical care environments has been revealed.[12] Failing to understand this cohesive view of a care team in a variety of settings risks a focus on the distant site that narrowly prescribes a solution certain to be deemed insufficient in today's health care environment. As the complexity of care increases for the critically ill patient, the necessity of a collaborative care team at the hub and spoke sites becomes more apparent.

TeleICU staffing models vary in the number of nurses and physicians to patients or beds. This variability depends on the workflow and support provided, resources available, and initiatives to control the cost of the TeleICU program.[3] Staffing structures should be established, and then evolve, based on the needs of the intensive care units (ICUs) that are supported by the TeleICU. These needs may differ among various ICUs and can be dynamic over shifts, suggesting that TeleICU staffing might look quite different overnight or over the weekend in comparison with a daytime shift.

According to Kahn and colleagues,[13] there are 4 major ways that TeleICU teams provide services: (1) monitor for physiologic deterioration, (2) diffusion of evidence-based practice, (3) expert advice and guidance, and (4) collecting, auditing, analyzing, and disseminating quality performance data. TeleICU staffing and workflows will differ based on the makeup of the bedside team. For example, in ICUs that lack intensivists on site, having around-the-clock presence of intensivists in the TeleICU to support evidence-based care decisions can improve patient outcomes. The TeleICU may augment intensivist and/or the advanced practice provider (APP) presence in the ICU to assist with managing multiple simultaneous demands or to provide support when the intensivist is not present. Intensivist presence in the TeleICU might not be around-the-clock; they may be present in higher-demand periods, and their workflows might call for them to advise and defer to the bedside team consistently. Technology capabilities and compatibilities and access to various software programs used in patient management will also impact team structure to a significant extent.

TeleICU TEAM MEMBERS

Most TeleICU clinical teams consist of a group of expert critical care nurses working with 1 or more physicians (generally intensivists) to support the care of critically ill and injured patients regardless of the patient's (and potentially the clinician's) location.[3,14,15] Some TeleICUs also use other disciplines, such as nurse practitioners, physician assistants, collectively referred to as APPs, as well as pharmacists and others.[3,14] Nonclinical support roles such as data assistant, clerical support, technical support, and quality and reporting analysts can round out the TeleICU team. Some of these variations will be discussed later in this article. Although this article will focus on clinical roles, the nonclinical positions are key to optimizing the role of the clinicians and their ability to function at the top of their license by providing clerical, triage, and data collection, analysis, and reporting support.[16]

In the intensivist-driven model, the critical care physician lies at the center of the team.[10] The intensivist relies on the TeleICU team members to provide key clinical information to alert them to proactively identify trends of deterioration before the impending clinical decline or patient cardiopulmonary arrest. In the TeleICU the intensivist may be responsible for the surveillance and management of upward of 100 to 250 patients.[3] At a Massachusetts academic health system, the TeleICU is staffed round the clock with intensivists who serve a primary role in managing the flow of patients into and out of the ICUs, along with providing critical care services and general supervision for APPs and residents when the managing intensivist is not available.[17] Tele-intensivist staffing ranges from 12 to 24 hours per day, depending on program design and/or need for services.[3]

The contributions and roles of APPs in the critical care workforce have been described in the literature.[18] Several organizations have integrated APP roles into their TeleICU. In these roles, Tele-APPs assess and evaluate patients using remote audio-video technologies, converse with families, provide consultation for bedside nurses, ensure adherence to best practices, and participate in care coordination and the management of unstable patients. The APP role can be invaluable in providing additional support to the tele-intensivist during high volume times in the hub.

The TeleICU nurse is usually responsible for 30 or more patients depending on the environment, level, and type of service being provided to the bedside, supporting technology, and other enabling capabilities.[3,19] The TeleICU nurse provides support to the TeleICU intensivist and to the bedside team.[2] A key function of the TeleICU nurse is to conduct ongoing reviews of large amounts of information to support the assessment and decision-making process for individual and populations of patients.[2] This function has been described as surveillance and supports the capturing, analyzing, and dissemination of relevant and clinically significant data.[19] Bedside assistance can be accomplished through support of initiatives such as assuring sedation vacations, surveying for appropriate sedation levels in ventilated patients, monitoring for the use of evidence-based best practices, or by acting as a mentor for novice ICU bedside nurses.[19] As described above, the role of the TeleICU nurse is determined by the need of the collaborative care team in caring for each site's patients.

Other clinical roles present in some TeleICUs, such as pharmacists and respiratory therapists, provide important services. For example, the pharmacist's expertise can be applied to manage vasopressors, anticoagulation medications, or deep vein thrombosis prophylaxis dosing. They may make recommendations for antibiotic de-escalation, or alert care team members to potential drug interactions as new medications are ordered. A study at a Massachusetts-based TeleICU demonstrated that pharmacists on the night shift could increase compliance with ICU sedation guidelines and extend the benefits provided by the daytime pharmacy team.[20] In Wisconsin, a TeleICU demonstrated that implementation of a remote ICU pharmacy service resulted in the provision of consistent pharmaceutical care, while minimizing costs at 13 hospitals.[21] A structured approach to glycemic control by TeleICU pharmacists at a large health system covering North and South Carolina resulted in tighter glycemic control in adult ICU patients without increasing rates of hypoglycemia.[22]

In recognizing the benefit of the pharmacist to the TeleICU team, one can begin to imagine roles for other disciplines. For example, respiratory therapists have been added to the clinical team of an independent national TeleICU provider to assist the team in the management of high-risk patients. Kacmarek[23] described that the role of the respiratory therapist in the management of mechanically ventilated patients has become paramount to providing evidence-based care of intubated patients. Kacmarek went on to describe that respiratory therapists can inform appropriate decision making related to initiation and adjustment of ventilator management, disease-specific management, analysis of ventilator waveforms, monitoring of mechanical ventilation and airway management, and assessment of diagnostic tests (laboratory and basic chest radiograph interpretation) and medication management.

GETTING TEAMS TO WORK TOGETHER: THE SYNERGY MODEL

Regardless of the specifics of team structure, some core principles must be overlaid to assure the team works effectively. The AACN TeleICU Taskforce describes how the Synergy Model for Patient Care provides a framework to enhance patient care and outcomes by matching patient characteristics/needs with nurse skill and competency.[2] AACN HWE provides criteria and standards for creating and sustaining optimal work atmospheres.[24] The Relational Coordination theoretic foundation focuses on key relationship dimensions of shared goals, shared knowledge, and mutual respect.[25] Along with the models described above, the theoretic foundation is provided that is especially relevant to TeleICU nursing practice and can be applied to all disciplines working in the TeleICU center (**Fig. 1**).[2] Clinical practice, skilled communication, collaborative relationships, and optimized technology are all characteristics that work interdependently to maintain a synergistic environment supporting the staff and the patient.[2] These interdependencies should be considered when developing workflows.[24]

COMMUNICATION IS KEY

If fee-for-service structures are to transform into a value-based oriented health care system, improved communication and true collaboration seem particularly necessary to achieve the goal of patient-focused care.[26] Communication plays a critical role in building successful teams, and patterns of communication were found to be the most important predictor of a team's success.[25] The communication between technology and the clinicians, both at the bedside and in the TeleICU, rely on the electronic medical record and various interfaces to access and track data relevant to the care of the patient. The TeleICU clinicians must use the data to forecast what may happen,

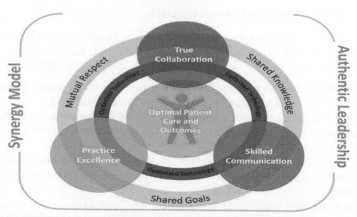

Fig. 1. AACN TeleICU nursing practice model. (*From* American Association of Critical-Care Nurses. AACN TeleICU Nursing Practice Model. AACN Tele-ICU Nursing Practice: An Expert Consensus Statement Supporting High Acuity, Progressive and Critical Care. Figure 1. Aliso Viejo (CA): American Association of Critical-Care Nurses. ©2018 by AACN. All rights reserved. Used with permission.)

design an appropriate plan in response, and then communicate those recommendations to their bedside counterparts. Communication between all the care providers must be clear and of high quality to achieve situational awareness.

Gittell described the Relational Coordination Model in which teams have shared goals, shared knowledge, and mutual respect. This leads to high-frequency communication that promotes quality collaboration resulting in patient safety and improved outcomes.[25] When there are problems or breakdowns between clinicians, the result may include preventable patient harm. The Joint Commission has found that communication issues are the most common root cause of sentinel events (serious and preventable patient harm incidents).[27]

The use of audio-visual technology as a communication tool places the remote care provider (physician, nurse, pharmacist, or APP) virtually at the bedside for visual and verbal communication and allows face-to-face dialog during the delivery of health care services.[5] A recent study by Kahn and colleagues[13] identified 3 domains as being key determinants of effective TeleICU teams in delivering improved clinical outcomes:

- Leadership: how organizational managers (ICU, TeleICU, and hospital system) make decisions about the role and reach of telemedicine.
- Perceived value: perceptions among front-line care providers about the ability of telemedicine to meaningfully improve clinical outcomes (including expectations of availability, understanding of operations, interpersonal relationships, and staff satisfaction).
- Organizational characteristics: features of the hub or distant and origin or spoke care sites that govern how remote clinical care is provided and received (such as staffing models and engagement protocols).

Kahn and colleagues[13] go on to say that programs that delivered decreases in risk-adjusted mortality after the implementation of TeleICU care tended to perform care activities in ways that were observed to be appropriate, responsive, consistent, and integrated with bedside workflows. This further validates a holistic view of the ICU team as consisting of both in-hospital and TeleICU personnel, and supports the significant emphasis on extensive communication within the team that is detailed above.

VARYING INTENSIVE CARE UNIT ENVIRONMENTS

The nature of origin care sites can differ dramatically, regardless of whether all ICUs are within a single system and especially if they are not. Key considerations that can affect the makeup of the TeleICU team include, but are not limited to

- The coverage and range of critical care expertise at the hospitals being served
- Hospital type: community or tertiary, teaching or nonteaching
- Types of ICUs to be covered and the concomitant bedside intensivist staff model
- Variations in coverage based on time of day, day of week, and/or hours of presence of intensivists at the bedside
- Whether the TeleICU is "within system" (ie, serving only hospitals within the same health system) or "trans-system" (ie, serving a range of independent and system hospitals)
- The technological capabilities that support the TeleICU
- The resources available to both the TeleICU program and each of the hospitals it serves (as scale increases, measured as number of beds, eg, additional resources or specialties, can be justified)

These factors should drive decisions related to structure, services, and team composition. The design of the TeleICU program should target the consistent delivery of high-quality care for all patients regardless of these or other variations, as measured by acuity-adjusted patient clinical outcomes, achievement of best practices, and operational considerations such as affordability and efficiency.

Most TeleICU centers begin as health system-level critical care initiatives. However, some TeleICUs serve hospitals in multiple health systems as well as individual, independent hospitals. One independent telemedicine provider, for example, was established specifically to provide TeleICU care to nonaffiliated hospitals and now supports over 75 independent and health system hospitals. In some situations, the TeleICU team augments intensivists and other critical care specialists within the hospital, whereas in others it provides the only critical care specialization.

Similarly, a large 23-hospital health system in New York has avoided a "one size fits all approach." By beginning with data collection, it imparted the technology and care model only where there was either demonstrated need based on APACHE (Acute Physiology and Chronic Health Evaluation—a standardized, risk-adjusted, severity of illness tool for ICU patients) score results or where there was expressed desire and need. Because every unit (even within the same hospital) had a different culture and staffing model, the approach to roll out and use of TeleICU was customized. This was not to say there were not standard components to be included in each new activation, but allowing key stakeholders to decide how and where this technology is implemented was essential to adaptation. In its tertiary hospitals with multiple critical care units, some units may have TeleICU coverage and others may not, depending on need and desire as described above. In other multi-ICU sites, all units may have TeleICU coverage. However, data collection surrounding outcomes is done uniformly in all units.

For some of the health system's community hospitals, the TeleICU becomes the main source of oversight starting in the late afternoon hours into the early morning. During this time there must be an APP available at the bedside capable of being the "hands" of the TeleICU intensivist. Because of the shortage of intensivists and location of some of the community hospitals, this combined staffing matrix is used differently at varying times of the day. However, what is clear is the ability of the TeleICU to support APPs at the bedside when an intensivist is not or cannot be present.

A health system located in Georgia was infused with a multimillion-dollar grant from the Centers for Medicare and Medicaid Services (CMS) in 2012 to launch a TeleICU program to support ICUs throughout Georgia.[28] This program is now providing night-time services to patients in Atlanta from Perth, Australia. This project was implemented to reduce clinician burn-out associated with working night shifts. According to a report by the CMS, the program has demonstrated reductions in the need for institutional postacute care after an ICU stay, a 2.1 percentage point decrease in 60-day readmission rates and a reduction in average spending of $1486 per 60-day episode yielding $4.6 million in Medicare savings. This health system uses APPs at the bedside supported by the TeleICU intensivists and nurses. APPs are engaged in the process of developing their role according to their scope of practice and based on the needs and perceptions of TeleICU and ICU staff.[29] APPs have the option of participating in a postgraduate residency program that has been accredited by the American Nurses Credentialing Center[30]

The aforementioned Massachusetts system has demonstrated and reported in the literature both outcome and financial benefits to using a 24/7 intensivist and APP model in its TeleICU.[17,31] Critical care nurses do not cover shifts in the TeleICU but do work collaboratively with the TeleICU providers. As mentioned previously, its Tele-ICU team serves a role in managing flow into and out of the 7 ICUs at the academic medical center. It also works with affiliated and managed care partner hospitals to provide high-level surveillance and critical care consultation services to keep patients at their home hospital when appropriate.[32]

POTENTIAL TEAM EXTENSIONS

Recently, there has been a move to include other clinical capacities in the TeleICU team. Ancillary support positions are implemented in specific TeleICUs when resources and demonstrated need exist. These positions can augment and leverage the capability of the TeleICU team and may include pharmacy, respiratory therapy, dieticians or any other position for which a need to support the bedside team can be demonstrated and financially justified. Using this core concept to leverage expertise can be highly effective in creating a systematic approach to critical care across health systems as well as across the country.

ONE OR MULTIPLE HUB SITES?

The TeleICU typically relies on centrally colocated teams, bringing all the skills into a single collaborative environment to provide care to the multiple spoke hospitals. Colocating teams in 1 place is cost-effective and creates the basis for an efficient and standardized model. However, it also introduces significant staffing risk, because all the necessary skilled TeleICU staff must be sourced in a single marketplace, which might be fraught with short supply or high competitive intensity. As an alternative, the ability to flexibly extend beyond the physical bounds of the TeleICU center and hospital can yield tremendous benefits. For example, the ability to coordinate care across multiple TeleICU centers enables recruitment of critical skills in diverse locations and can thus serve to mitigate these key risks of a single center.

In the recent merger of 2 large Midwest health systems to become a single entity, where each system has a mature TeleICU hub, a decision has been made to retain the 2 hub sites while planning to integrate and standardize the care delivery model. The benefit of this decision allows for recruitment of clinicians in both states (Illinois and Wisconsin). This widens the depth and breadth of the pool of available expertise (medical, pulmonary, surgical, trauma, neuro, anesthesia, and cardiovascular) from which to pull while establishing standard workflows in both hubs. This will assure consistency of care delivery regardless of the state from which the care is provided. The hub teams can be leveraged through cross-state licensing to establish patient assignments that may mix care between ICUs in both states to establish appropriate TeleICU workloads. In a similar example, the largest independent TeleICU care provider discussed earlier now uses a network of 9 care centers to support TeleICU care to hospitals nationwide. This enables multi-site recruiting and leverages time zone differences to mitigate local staffing risk and provide extensive system redundancy and resilience.

ADDITIONAL USES OF THE TeleICU TEAM/TECHNOLOGY

As discussed throughout, critical care is ever evolving, as are the roles and functions of the clinicians in this environment. As one considers the TeleICU team and its ability to support the interdisciplinary team, some additional methods of use could be considered as follows.

As Mentors

The use of expert TeleICU nurses to support decision making and translation of evidence-based practice has been described in the literature.[3,16,19] Experienced clinicians in the TeleICU can also be leveraged to mentor and support novice ICU clinicians. In the nursing arena, some approaches that have been taken to accomplish this include post bedside orientation mentoring and developing critical thinking skills using the TeleICU technology for novice ICU registered nurses (RNs). In one system's mentoring program, specific program objectives, structure, implementation, and evaluation are developed.[33] This allows each bedside RN who participates to feel supported in progressing from a novice nurse to an advanced beginner.

In another implementation of a critical thinking development program, new ICU RNs were given case scenarios, with the TeleICU technology integrated via screenshots to give examples of vital sign deterioration, trending in laboratories, and so forth. This allowed the novice RNs to evaluate actual patient data when making clinical care decisions. The benefit to the TeleICU in acting as the mentor is 2-fold:

1. The experienced TeleICU RN can share his or her expertise and knowledge, giving a sense of meaning to their work beyond the remote monitoring of patients; and
2. The critical relationship between caregivers on both sides of the camera, so vital to open communication and integration of the TeleICU into the ICU care team, is established and nurtured.[34,35]

TeleICU teams can offer benefits related to mentoring of residents and APPs with TeleICU intensivist oversight and remote participation in ICU sign-out.[35] During the night shift in 1 health system located in Delaware, physician assistants call the TeleICU intensivist in Illinois to discuss all new admissions and rapid response team patients. This case review provides guidance on patient management and establishes the plan of care overnight. As a side benefit to this structure for overnight partnership, these discussions and case presentations are conducted with an awake and alert TeleICU intensivist. Further, the bedside attending physician is afforded much-needed sleep, which preserves his or her sleep architecture. These models leverage the scarce resource of an attending intensivist to provide "at the end of a phone line" consultation for hundreds of patients who may be hundreds of miles away.[36] These factors, in combination, help prevent bedside physician burn-out while augmenting the development of the APPs and residents.

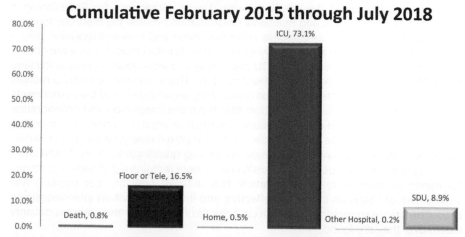

Fig. 2. eMobile cart percent by unit discharge location. (*Courtesy of* Advocate Health Care eICU.)

Real-time mentorship can extend to a variety of health care roles through experiential learning in the live TeleICU environment. Further, exposure to such programs can provide insight into the ever-changing models of patient care. Nursing students and other health care professionals in training are afforded an opportunity to glimpse their future career opportunities as experienced clinicians.

In Other Care Settings

Several TeleICU teams have extended their services in the emergency department (ED). Critical care experts in the TeleICU work with fellow team members to provide care to ICU boarders in the ED. A TeleICU in Illinois has demonstrated that, through the deployment of the TeleICU technology in the ED, about 30% of the time, patients can be admitted to a less acute level of care (floor/tele or stepdown unit) by the time a bed becomes available (**Fig. 2**). Team members working together to provide the right care at the right time results in both patient and staff satisfaction, as well as cost savings to the hospital. Other care settings for which the TeleICU technology has been leveraged include postanesthesia care units, behavioral health, disaster response, high-risk obstetrics, and to assist in timely management of patients who have had a stroke.[37]

SUMMARY

This article has discussed a framework within which to evaluate the appropriate composition and deployment of a TeleICU team in support of critically ill patients. The essential team structure combines expert clinical knowledge from both the TeleICU and bedside and is leveraged in a way that is flexible based on unit needs. This agility allows support that can be adapted to the individual needs of the critical care environment. Several factors must be considered when making this decision, not least of which is a method to establish consistent communication and subsequently, effective workflows to impact patient outcomes. Each organization must consider its resources (both human and financial) as well as culture and patient population needs when establishing an infrastructure.

The core principles of the AACN Synergy Model, Standards for Establishing a Healthy Work Environment and Relational Coordination provide the theoretic foundation of critical care practice. Effective communication and true collaboration play a critical role in both quality and safety when using the TeleICU model. There are opportunities to explore the effect of TeleICU mentoring and education on critical thinking capabilities of the novice nurse and other providers. There are varying TeleICU models that may be deployed depending on the goals of the organization and the components of the clinical team. Research has shown that the more integration and collaboration between the TeleICU and ICU, the greater the positive impact on patient outcomes.

TeleICU continues to be a new frontier for critical care delivery, which allows expertise to be available in a range of hospitals, enhancing quality care nationally and internationally. After nearly 2 decades of TeleICU use, there remains significant opportunity for expansion and evolution. This article has outlined how the composition and deployment of TeleICUs can be an effective and integral part of an interdisciplinary critical care team supporting the health care needs of vulnerable and complex patients where ever they are found.

REFERENCES

1. American Telemedicine Association. About Telemedicine: Q&A; 2016. Available at: http://www.americantelemed.org/main/about/telehealth-faqs-. Accessed February 27, 2017.
2. American Association of Critical Care Nurses (AACN) TeleICU Task Force. AACN TeleICU nursing practice: an expert consensus statement supporting high acuity, progressive and critical care. Aliso Viejo (CA): AACN; 2018.
3. Davis TM, Barden C, Dean S, et al. American telemedicine association guidelines for TeleICU operations. Telemed J E Health 2016;22:971–80.
4. Thomas L, Capistrant G. State telemedicine gaps analysis: coverage & reimbursement. Washington, DC: American Telemedicine Association; 2017.
5. Reynolds HN, Bander J, McCarthy M. Different systems and formats for tele-ICU coverage: designing a tele-ICU system to optimize functionality and investment. Crit Care Nurs Q 2012;35:364–77.
6. Dayal P, Hojman NM, Kissee JL, et al. Impact of telemedicine on severity of illness and outcomes among children transferred from referring emergency departments to a children's hospital PICU. Pediatr Crit Care Med 2016;17:516–21.
7. Ellenby MS, Marcin JP. The role of telemedicine in pediatric critical care. Crit Care Clin 2015;31:275–90.
8. Rogove H. How to develop a tele-ICU model? Crit Care Nurs Q 2012;35:357–63.
9. Goran SF. A new view: tele-intensive care unit competencies. Crit Care Nurse 2011;31:17–29.
10. Lilly CM, Zubrow MT, Kempner KM, et al. Critical care telemedicine: evolution and state of the art. Crit Care Med 2014;42:2429–36.
11. Rosenfeld BA, Dorman T, Breslow MJ, et al. Intensive care unit telemedicine: alternate paradigm for providing continuous intensivist care. Crit Care Med 2000;28:3925–31.
12. Kim MM, Barnato AE, Angus DC, et al. The effect of multidisciplinary care teams on intensive care unit mortality. Arch Intern Med 2010;170:369–76.
13. Kahn JM, Rak KJ, Kuza CC, et al. Determinants of intensive care unit telemedicine effectiveness: an ethnographic study. Am J Respir Crit Care Med 2018. https://doi.org/10.1164/rccm.201802-0259OC.

14. Udeh C, Udeh B, Rahman N, et al. Telemedicine/virtual ICU: where are we and where are we going? Methodist Debakey Cardiovasc J 2018;14:126–33.
15. Kahn JM, Le TQ, Barnato AE, et al. ICU telemedicine and critical care mortality: a national effectiveness study. Med Care 2016;54:319–25.
16. Goran SF. A second set of eyes: an introduction to Tele-ICU. Crit Care Nurse 2010;30:46–55.
17. Lilly CM, Motzkus C, Rincon T, et al. ICU telemedicine program financial outcomes. Chest 2017;151:286–97.
18. Buchman T, Boyle W, Beyatte M. Shaping the next critical care workforce. In: Kleinpell RM, Boyle WA, Buchman TG, editors. Integrating nurse practitioners & physician assistants into the ICU: strategies for optimizing contributions to care. Mount Prospect (IL): Society of Critical Care Medicine; 2012.
19. Rincon TA, Henneman E. An introduction to nursing surveillance in the tele-ICU. Nurs Crit Care 2018;13:42–6.
20. Forni A, Skehan N, Hartman CA, et al. Evaluation of the impact of a tele-ICU pharmacist on the management of sedation in critically ill mechanically ventilated patients. Ann Pharmacother 2010;44:432–8.
21. Meidl TM, Woller TW, Iglar AM, et al. Implementation of pharmacy services in a telemedicine intensive care unit. Am J Health Syst Pharm 2008;65:1464–9.
22. Everhart S, Kosmisky D, Karvetski C, et al. Tele-ICU Pharmacist Impact on Glycemic Control Across a Large Healthcare System. 2016 ASHP Best Practice Award; 2016. Available at: https://www.ashp.org/About-ASHP. Accessed November 12, 2018.
23. Kacmarek RM. Mechanical ventilation competencies of the respiratory therapist in 2015 and beyond. Respir Care 2013;58:1087–96.
24. American Association of Critical Care Nurses (AACN). AACN standards for establishing and maintaining healthy work environments. Aliso Viejo (CA): AACN; 2016.
25. Gittell JH, Godfrey M, Thistlethwaite J. Interprofessional collaborative practice and relational coordination: improving healthcare through relationships. J Interprof Care 2013;27:210–3.
26. McCauley K, Irwin RS. Changing the work environment in intensive care units to achieve patient-focused care: the time has come. Am J Crit Care 2006;15:541–8.
27. Patient Safety Network (PSNet). Communication Between Clinicians. Patient Safety Primer; 2018. Available at: https://psnet.ahrq.gov/primers/primer/26/Communication-Between-Clinicians. Accessed November 12, 2018.
28. Woodruff Health Sciences Center. Emory cares for ICU patients remotely, turning 'night into day' from Australia. Emory News Center; 2018. Available at: https://news.emory.edu/stories/2018/05/buchman-hiddleson_eicu_perth_australia/index.html. Accessed November 12, 2018.
29. Leventhal R. Emory healthcare saves $4.6M with tele-ICU program. Healthcare Informatics; 2017. Available at: https://www.healthcare-informatics.com/news-item/telemedicine/emory-healthcare-saves-46m-tele-icu-program. Accessed November 12, 2018.
30. American Nurses Credentialing Center (ANCC). Emory critical care center nurse practitioner residency program: gaining accreditation to better support nurse practitioners. Silver Spring (MD): ANCC; 2015.
31. Lilly C, Cody S, Zhao H, et al. Hospital mortality, length of stay, and preventable complications among critically ill patients before and after tele-ICU reengineering of critical care processes. JAMA 2011;305:E1–9.

32. New England Healthcare Institute and Massachusetts Technology Collaborative. Tele-ICUs: remote management in intensive care units. Cambridge (MA): New England Healthcare Institute (NEHI); 2007. p. 1–37.

33. Brindise T, Baker MP, Juarez P. Development of a tele-ICU postorientation support program for bedside nurses. Crit Care Nurse 2015;35:e8–16.

34. Mullen-Fortino M, DiMartino J, Entrikin L, et al. Bedside nurses' perceptions of intensive care unit telemedicine. Am J Crit Care 2012;21:24–31 [quiz: 2].

35. Venditti A, Ronk C, Kopenhaver T, et al. Tele-ICU "Myth Busters". AACN Adv Crit Care 2012;23:302–11.

36. Goran SF, Mullen-Fortino M. Partnership for a healthy work environment: tele-ICU/ICU collaborative. AACN Adv Crit Care 2012;23:289–301.

37. Healthcare P. eICU program: Telehealth for the intensive care unit. Philips Enterprise telehealth; 2017. Available at: https://www.usa.philips.com/healthcare/product/HCNOCTN503/eicu-program-telehealth-for-the-intensive-care-unit. Accessed October 21, 2017.

Tele-ICU Technologies

Vitaly Herasevich, MD, PhD, FCCM[a],*, Sanjay Subramanian, MD, MMM[b]

KEYWORDS

- Telemedicine • Intensive care unit • Tele-ICU • eICU

KEY POINTS

- Information technologies today can be effective for supporting Tele-ICU systems.
- Privacy and security of electronic health information is an important component of a Tele-ICU system.
- A limited number of Tele-ICU vendors exist in the market.
- The information contained in this article is not intended to serve as technical and legal advice. When building a Tele-ICU program readers are encouraged to seek additional detailed technical and legal guidance to supplement the information contained below.

INTRODUCTION

In general population terms, "telemedicine" is often interchangeably used with term "telehealth." However, telemedicine and especially Tele-ICU are narrower and more specific uses of telehealth technologies. The Agency for Healthcare Research and Quality definition of telehealth is "the use of telecommunications technologies to deliver health-related services and information that support patient care, administrative activities, and health education.[1]" The American Telemedicine Association defines telemedicine as "the use of medical information, exchanged from one site to another via electronic communications, to improve patients' health status.[2]"

The telehealth services can broadly include technologies that are not used exclusively for telemedicine. Web-based patient e-health services such as health/patient Internet portals and consumer medical and health information resources are great examples of telehealth services in general. However, other modes of communication such as audio-only (telephone) or written communication (e-mail, messengers, fax) are generally not considered as telemedicine.

Disclosure Statement: The authors have no relevant commercial or financial conflicts of interest.

[a] Department of Anesthesiology and Perioperative Medicine, Division of Critical Care, Mayo Clinic, 200 First Street Southwest, Rochester, MN 55905, USA; [b] Department of Anesthesiology, Division of Critical Care, Washington University in St. Louis, PO Box 8054, 660 South Euclid Avenue, St Louis, MO 63110, USA
* Corresponding author.
E-mail address: vitaly@mayo.edu

Crit Care Clin 35 (2019) 427–438
https://doi.org/10.1016/j.ccc.2019.02.009
0749-0704/19/© 2019 Elsevier Inc. All rights reserved.

criticalcare.theclinics.com

The distinguishing feature that qualifies remote health services as telemedicine is the presence of a real-time audiovisual communication tool that connects providers and patients across geographies. The second feature of telemedicine is the use of "store-and-forward" technologies (in most cases electronic medical records [EMRs] at patient location) that collect patient's clinical data such as notes, laboratory values, and images, and transmit the same to remote clinicians. In addition, Tele-ICU may include real-time remote patient-monitoring tools and ability to place remote orders using Computerized Provider Order Entry (CPOE).

In recent years, a drastic increase in the use mobile wireless technologies (mHealth) for such purposes has been observed. Usage of such technologies also could qualify as telemedicine. In general telemedicine and telehealth have complementary goals and synergistic activities.

HISTORY AND EVOLVING TECHNOLOGY OF TELEMEDICINE IN THE INTENSIVE CARE UNIT

Telemedicine technology was imagined by people even before the actual technological capability existed. The *Radio News* magazine cover in April 1924 published a system that in fact looks like a modern telemedicine station. (Commercial television was not introduced at that time. However, the first real television signal transmission happened only in 1927 after that picture was published. Vladimir K. Zworykin applied for an electronic television patent in 1923, but his prototype did not work until 1934.)

The Royal Flying Doctor Service in Australia is the longest running telemedicine provider in the world, which started by using a pedal-powered generator connected to a transceiver for Morse code. In the mid-1930s, voice radio was adopted.[3] In the 1960s, the US Department of Defense, The National Aeronautics and Space Administration (NASA), and the Health and Human Sciences Department invested in telemedicine research. NASA involvement in telemedicine was applied in the public setting during earthquakes in Mexico City 1985 and Armenia in 1988.[4] Most of the telemedicine projects between 1960 and 1980, mostly grants and trial projects, failed because of telecommunication costs and nonavailability of advanced technologies. The first commercial telemedicine system used landline telephone lines and was developed by MedPhone Corporation in 1989. The transtelephonic defibrillator/monitor was a US Food and Drug Administration (FDA)-approved interactive communication system to diagnose and treat patients requiring cardiac resuscitation defibrillation remotely.

A visual distant link for the care of critically ill patients reported in 1977,[5] in which 2-way audiovisual connection between a small private hospital and a large university medical center, was used to provide daily consultations by an intensivist. Another use of telemedicine in critical care as an intermittent consultative device was reported in 1982.[6] For 18 months, 395 patients in the intensive care unit (ICU) in a 100-bed hospital received a telemedicine "visit" using television consultation from university-based critical care physicians with no on-site intensivist.

In 1997, staff at a hospital affiliated with John Hopkins performed a study in surgical ICU using video conferencing equipment connecting to intensivists' homes. This enabled direct visualization and communication to patients and on-site caregivers on an intermittent basis. Bedside data from Spacelabs, monitors were transmitted in real-time through a telephone system. In addition, a telephone terminal-emulation system was used to access laboratory data. As the ICU had no EMRs, all documentation was scanned and transmitted to the intensivist digitally.[7] The first Tele-ICU in the United States using modern technologies to monitor and treat ICU patients remotely was implemented in 2000 in Sentara Hospital, Norfolk, Virginia. As technologies were expensive during that time, it was difficult to justify the investment in Tele-ICU.

Broader acceptance of Tele-ICU occurred after 2004 when an article published by John Hopkins University showed an improvement in ICU and hospital mortality using a Tele-ICU care model.[8] The Tele-ICU solution used in that study (VISICU) is still the dominant platform for Tele-ICU programs. Between 2003 and 2010 the number of hospitals using Tele-ICU increased from 16 to 213.[9] As of 2011, 41 Tele-ICU command centers ("hubs") cover 249 hospitals nationwide.[10]

Advances in information and computing technologies have triggered greater affordability and accessibility of telemedicine tools. Teams of ICU providers from 1 Tele-ICU hub can provide care for up to 150 ICU patients across multiple hospitals.[11] However, the technical structure of today's Tele-ICU solution is still fundamentally not different from 20 years ago in terms of basic organizational structure and functionality.

TELE-ICU TECHNOLOGY

In recent decades, technologies required for Tele-ICU programs have reached a point of cost-efficiency mostly because data transmission moved from dedicated optical cable networks to virtual private networks over public Internet.[12] The critical requirement for a Tele-ICU program is reliable communication between the Tele-ICU team (hub) and the remote ICU.

ICUs have a unique workflow and patient characteristics that are reflected in the technology used. Understanding types of care delivery models and organizational characteristics will help define the technology needs for Tele-ICU platforms.

From an organizational perspective Tele-ICU services have 2 different types of administrative structure:

- Networked programs. The main characteristic here is a single hub center that provides Tele-ICU services for multiple locations. For example, large academic metropolitan hospitals that offer a service to surrounding small rural hospitals.
- Point-to-point program. The main characteristic is that smaller or understaffed hospitals outsource medical care to specialists at a large central health care facility usually within the same health system.

The monitoring center (hub) is staffed and operationalized by physician-intensivists, advanced practice providers (APP), registered nurses (RNs), and administrative and technical support staff.

The type of care delivery models for Tele-ICU, in turn, drives the development of technological solutions. Whereas most existing Tele-ICU systems are based on a design with a centralized support center and continuous care model, care delivery models can be divided into 4 common types:

- Continuous care model. Remote monitoring of distant ICUs on 24/7 continuous basis. This model uses an operational center staffed by a team of ICU physicians, APPs, and RNs. It has high readability connections with backup and IT professional support.
- Episodic care model. Remote care that has an intermittent schedule (daily rounds, shift changes) or unscheduled connection sessions between patient and provider, only provider to provider, or both.
- Responsive care model. Reactive, episodic care occurs when a remote consultation is prompted by an alarm or telephone call.

- Remote patient monitoring. The remote health care provider uses telemetry devices to remotely collect and send data to their monitoring station for interpretation.

Depending on the particular Tele-ICU program, the hardware and software configuration could be different, but, in general modalities for delivering Tele-ICU, are the following:

- Real-time/live (synchronous): a 2-way audiovisual link between a patient and a remote clinician
- Store-and-forward (asynchronous): transmission of a recorded health history to a health practitioner, usually a physician or APP. This could also include the use of CPOE
- Remote patient monitoring: the use of connected electronic tools, such as bedside monitors, to transfer real-time data from the patient location to a telemedicine provider in another location, usually by an RN

HARDWARE AND SOFTWARE SPECIFICATIONS

There are many technological requirements for establishing a Tele-ICU center to practice meaningful and safe care delivery. Technology lifecycle is very short, and many technologies have become obsolete over the years and only remain as of historical interest.

Also typical technological solutions are vendor dependent.

Network or Communication Link

The essential technical requirement is a secure high-speed communication line with backup. This was, in fact, a technological barrier to adoption of Tele-ICU because earlier systems used dedicated cables and fiber optic links that were expensive to establish and maintain. The widely accessible telephone modem connections and Integrated Services Digital Network line were not sufficient to transmit real-time data such as video and audio with acceptable quality. However, currently available commercial broadband Internet networks are reliable and have adequate speed to support multiple Tele-ICU stations. In 2015, the Federal Communications Commission altered the definition of broadband by increasing the minimum download/upload speed from 4 Mbps/1 Mbps to 25 Mbps/3 Mbps.

Available network bandwidth is a limiting factor for live video quality. To overcome the bandwidth barrier, data compression protocols are applied to video and audio stream. Currently, the most common compression protocol is H.264/MPEG-4 AVC evolved from an H.323 standard. It has excellent video quality and preserves bandwidth by lower bit rates than previous standards. H.323 was introduced in 2003, the video surveillance industry adopted it first, and since then it has become the standard. The recommended bandwidth for a high-definition 1080p video at 30 frames per second rate is 1024 kbit per second. Network connection should include some overhead in bandwidth to accommodate multiple video/audio streams and other data such as EMRs, a Picture Archiving and Communication System (PACS), and bedside monitor feeds. Hospitals are likely to use a commercial Internet provider, and proper Quality of Service and configuration of the network is important to support multiple video feeds and other concurrent data transfers.

As well as commercial communication links, Virtual Private Network (VPN) protocols are used to secure communication. Backup communication is essential for the reliable operation of a Tele-ICU center, and a cellular network could be one such option.

Modern mobile networks, such as Long-Term Evolution, have sufficient bandwidth for transmitting high-quality videos. In terms of reliability, however, wired systems perform better in avoiding latency, dropouts, or loss of connectivity.

Computer Equipment

Presently, any modern office or EMR capable computer has enough computation power to run Tele-ICU software. Local information technology (IT) departments may prefer different vendors of PC-compatible computers. However, most software types used in the Tele-ICU setting are not Macintosh compatible. All equipment should be connected to a power network with an Uninterruptible Power Supply that can support sufficient time for computer operation until main power is restored. Emergency power electric generators can support Tele-ICU center operations for a prolonged time in case of disaster.

Computer/Display Monitors

The technology has moved entirely from the cathode-ray tube displays to "flat panel" liquid-crystal display. Large computer displays have since become affordable. Since the Tele-ICU operator spends the entire shift in front of computer monitors, a few characteristics are essential for high-quality displays.

- Size. The current 2019 standard logical minimum size of a single monitor is 24 inches. Some EMR vendors required this size to be "certified" for using their system. Larger 27-inch monitors, set up as a 6-monitor panel configuration, offers an even more attractive ergonomic display.
- Monitor resolution. Typical resolution of a modern monitor is 1920×1080 pixels. This is referred to as a high-definition screen and should be considered as a minimum for a modern setup. Recent advantages in monitoring technologies have introduced 4K monitors with 3840×2160 pixel resolution. Their resolution is double in each dimension. Technically the same screen has 4 times more pixels and visually the picture is crisper for the user. There are no clear advantages for such monitors for Tele-ICU setup except for the video quality and radiology/PACS viewing. Given the fast technological progress, such monitors could be considered a good investment. Another important parameter of monitors is the technology used in liquid-crystal display screens. It is recommended to use monitors built with in-plane switching (IPS) technology. IPS monitors have a wide view angle of 178°/178° compared with twisted nematic (TN) monitors. TN monitors have a narrow angle of view that would limit collaboration among multiple users. More modern vertical alignment monitors have better angles, but, however, are not superior to IPS display, especially with regard to color reproduction. The color depth of TN monitors is limited to 18 bit (262,144 colors), whereas a typical IPS monitor is capable of reproducing True color (24 bit) with 16 million colors. The photorealistic 30-bit monitor shows 1073 billion colors and can be recommended for all imaging applications.

Video Cameras

Earlier telemedicine systems used video teleconferencing equipment that offered high video quality. Polycom (now part of Plantronics) and Cisco Systems were the manufacturers often used in those setups. The company Lifesize introduced the first high-definition video conferencing system in 2005. These solutions could be used on portable carts that could be moved to any patient location. However, one of the standard technical guidelines for Tele-ICU is fixed high-quality cameras in the patient rooms. Ideally, cameras should have the pan-tilt-zoom capability, enabled with a microphone, speaker, and monitor for 2-way audio and video communication. The American Telemedicine Association (ATA) guidelines suggest a minimum of 640 × 360 pixel resolution at 30 frames per second video transmission. However, the current practical minimum standard should be at the level of high-definition video, with 1920 × 1080 pixel resolution recommended. With the introduction of 4K videos, modern and future Tele-ICU systems will have great benefit from higher-resolution cameras; however, such videos will require network channels with greater bandwidth.

Mobile Technologies

Although Tele-ICU often uses fixed in-room hardware, remote telemedicine carts or robots or mobile devices could be used for this purpose. For example, the FDA-cleared medical telepresence robot from InTouch has been used for Tele-ICU. This product is built in collaboration with iRobot, best known in the customer market for Roomba vacuum-cleaning robots.

Access to Core Electronic Medical Records

The EMR is a crucial component of telemedicine. Whereas a video communication link is an essential element of a Tele-ICU system, access to the entire patient record is required for accuracy and safety. There are no requirements from governing bodies on how to document a telemedicine encounter. However, it should be consistent, accurate, and timely, and should not be duplicative.[13] Access to core EMRs such as Epic or Cerner solutions is established through the same VPN communication link and is very much a standard feature. The EMRs usually integrate laboratory and pathology data, and include CPOE.

Access to Radiology and Other Residual Systems

PACS is traditionally a separate system within the suite of comprehensive EMR tools. Remote access to the PACS system is accomplished using the same approach as the core EMRs. Radiology images are typically heavy on data usage, and this should be accounted for while planning for bandwidth.

Tele-ICU Manager

This is a unique component of the Tele-ICU system that enables population management. Such a system allows the user to oversee the whole ICU unit and communicate concerns to the bedside providers. Usually, it has an acuity scoring system and an alerting component for physiologic deterioration. An example of such a system is the Philips eCareManager (**Fig. 1**).

Ancillary Devices

Whereas video and audio communication, and access to EMRs and bedside monitors, may be sufficient for an Tele-ICU encounter, the addition of medical devices could enhance the telemedicine experience to the next level. There is a variety of telemedicine-enabled equipment available on the market, including otoscopes, stethoscopes, ultrasounds probes, spirometers, and electrocardiograph equipment, which are FDA cleared.

Tele-ICU Call Button

A distinguishing feature of telemedicine solutions for ICU includes a call button used to initiate a telemedicine session on demand from the bedside with the

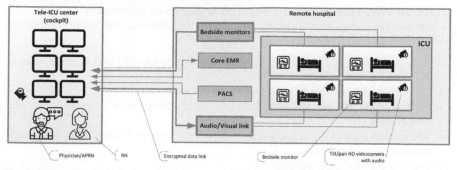

Fig. 1. Schematic technical outline of a comprehensive Tele-ICU system.

remote provider. It should be placed no more than 48 inches above the floor to meet the Americans with Disabilities Act of 1990 requirements. A phone with direct dial to Tele-ICU hub is required as backup communication.

REGULATIONS AND CYBERSECURITY

Privacy and security of electronic health information is a key component and requirement for any Tele-ICU system. The Health Insurance Portability and Accountability Act (HIPAA) of 1996 Privacy and Security Rules are to protect the privacy and security of individually identifiable health information. HIPAA rules pertains to any media format including paper or electronic.

1. The privacy standards set boundaries on the use of health information. They also provide safeguards that must be followed to protect the privacy of health information.

   Advances in the past decade in consumer-level video conferencing have encouraged the use of systems such as FaceTime, Whatsapp, and Skype for teleconsultations. However, not all of them are HIPAA compliant. Based on the HIPAA Security Rule published in the Federal Register on February 20, 2003 (45 CFR Parts 160, 162, and 164 Health Insurance Reform: Security Standards; Final Rule) the general requirements are[14]:

   - Ensure the confidentiality, integrity, and availability of all electronic protected health information (ePHI) the covered entity creates, receives, maintains, or transmits
   - Protect against any reasonably anticipated threats or hazards to the security or integrity of such information
   - Protect against any reasonably anticipated uses or disclosures of such information that are not permitted or required
   - Ensure compliance by the workforce

   For a software to be compliant with HIPAA, a Business Associate Agreement needs to be signed. That means all business associates sign contracts to make sure that all PHI is safeguarded by everyone who accesses the same.

2. The security standards require all health care providers to assess the risks to their information systems and to take appropriate steps to ensure the confidentiality, integrity, and availability of patient information.

There are 3 main categories of safeguards of electronic information.

Administrative safeguards establish standards, regulations, and specifications for health information security.

- They establish security management processes to identify and analyze risks to PHI
- Computer-use policies to enforce proper access
- Staff training to ensure knowledge of and compliance with policies and procedures
- Information access management policies to limit access PHI to the minimum limit required for patient care
- Backup plan for emergencies

Physical safeguards control physical access to facilities and computer systems by users.

- Access controls to facilities with computer systems for authorized personnel only such as the use of badges, locks, and alarms
- Computers secured against theft using cable locks
- Computer monitor privacy filters to guard against the unauthorized view of information

Technical safeguards include hardware, software, and other technologies that limit access to PHI.

- Access controls to restrict access to PHI by authorized personnel only
- Audit controls. Each episode of access to EMRs and Tele-ICU system should be documented, including details of time accessed, and the person accessing the system to provide a record for future auditing purposes
- Integrity controls to prevent improper EMR alteration or destruction
- Data transmission security to protect patient's information when transmitted over a computer network. Full encryption is another requirement for a HIPAA-compliant solution. All network traffic should be encrypted at least to 256-bit Advanced Encryption Standard level, and no intermediary should have access to encryption keys. The video and audio are transmitted using a secure peer-to-peer connection with no video storage

Since 2012, more low-cost, high-quality, telehealth-oriented HIPAA-compliant video telemedicine services have entered the market and could also be used for Tele-ICU solutions. VSee, Chiron Health, Secure Video, Zoom, Vidyo, and Doxy.me are some of the emerging players for video telemedicine solutions.

To protect patient information and organizational assets, strong cybersecurity practices are important. Cybersecurity is important for compliance with the HIPAA Security Rule and protects the confidentiality, integrity, and availability of EMR and Tele-ICU systems.

HEALTH INFORMATION TECHNOLOGY STANDARDS AND INTEROPERABILITY

The objective of interoperability in health IT is to connect the different elements of health care in the digital ecosystem and facilitate optimal networking and communications between them. Technical standards are necessary for maintaining quality and ensuring interoperability of health care data. Tele-ICU is a diverse system that connects many technological/software solutions across multiple health care organizations and integrates off-the-shelf hardware components and other software applications. Although these systems perform well, it can be challenging to add new functionalities and communicate with other telemedicine vendors. The Tele-ICU community still needs to define and develop telemedicine systems interoperability standards and specifications.

Interoperability standards are usually developed by industry and adopted by regulatory/legislative action (de jure standard), but sometimes standards are defined by acceptance and widespread adoption (de facto standard). Health data standards can be grouped into 2 big categories: transport and terminology standards. The Centers for Medicare & Medicaid Services, Office of the National Coordinator for Health IT, and FDA require the use of certain health IT standards such as X12, NCPDP, ICD, NDC, and CPT for Claims Transactions and NCPDP Standards for ePrescribing (**Table 1**).

Interoperability provides a framework and tools for clinical providers from differing locations, specialties, and organizations be able to work together to provide clinical care. Standards are essential and allow

- Exchange of information with other clinicians, and other health care and administrative organizations
- Adoption of new tools and software to existing systems with minimum effort and cost
- Ensuring integrity and confidentiality of PHI
- Use of a variety of technological infrastructure adopted across different clinical settings.

VENDORS AND TELE-ICU TECHNOLOGIES

Over recent decades the eCARE Manager (formerly VISICU) system from Philips has dominated the Tele-ICU market.[15] VISICU was founded as an independent spin-off company from John Hopkins University and in 2006 was acquired by Philips. They received FDA 510K approval of the Smart Alarms module and eCareManager, which collects, stores, and displays clinical data obtained from the EMRs, patient-monitoring systems, and ancillary systems connected through networks. The system was built using the VISICU ARGUS System and uses Axis Communications high-quality cameras.

There has been a growth of many companies offering many related telemedicine solutions, but none is close to Tele-ICU market penetration in the United States compared with Phillips. Telehealth InTouch software is category leader for Virtual Care in the "2018 Best in KLAS: Software & Services" however, its use as a Tele-ICU solution is not well documented in the literature.

One of the limiting factors in implementing a Tel-ICU solution is the technology costs, in particular Philips systems. Traditionally, they are offered as hardware-software closed systems. Because technology has evolved and become less expensive over time, we have observed an increase in "non-traditional" telemedicine vendors. Almost every EMR vendor such as Epic or GE Healthcare offer their own telemedicine solutions, in general by adding a video communication link on top of EMR software. However, these are on-demand telemedicine solutions and cannot be considered as Tele-ICU active patient-monitoring (APM) systems. FDA has guidance regarding differentiating APM from medical device data systems (MDDS). Devices (including software devices) used for APM must be FDA class II certified. MDDS is not intended to be used in connection with APM.[16,17] Moreover, the hospital would be in violation of the FDA ruling if uncertified cameras and monitoring equipment were used in acute decision making.[18] Currently, FDA class II certified

Table 1
Data exchange and terminology standards

Data exchange transport standards	
Health Level Seven (HL7)	Provides several standards for exchanging clinical data and is used as the basis for many exchange standards currently used in health IT. HL7 is the underlying basis for standards like FHIR and CDA
HL7 Clinical Document Architecture (CDA)	CDA: is an XML-based exchange model for clinical documents such as discharge summaries and progress notes
Fast Healthcare Interoperability Resources (FHIR)	Is an HL7-based draft standard. It would simplify the exchange of health information using modern Web-based application programming interface technology
X12	Provides a standard for the electronic exchange of business transactions-electronic data interchange including insurance industry's business activities
National Council for Prescription Drug Programs (NCPDP)	National standard for electronic health care transactions used in prescribing, dispensing, monitoring, managing, and paying for medications and pharmacy services
Digital Imaging and Communications in Medicine	The standard for the communication and management of medical imaging information and related data. It is used in PACS
Health care data terminology standards	
International Statistical Classification of Diseases (ICD)	Currently the 10th revision of the ICD. It is supported by the World Health Organization and contains codes for diseases, signs, and symptoms
Systematized Nomenclature of Medicine Clinical Terms (SNOMED CT)	SNOMED CT: provides comprehensive computerized clinical terminology covering clinical data for diseases, clinical findings, and procedures
Current Procedural Terminology (CPT) and Healthcare Common Procedure Coding System (HCPCS)	CPT is a code set maintained by the American Medical Association used to bill outpatient and office procedures. HCPCS is a set of CPT-based codes used for the Center for Medicare and Medicaid services billing
National Drug Code (NDC)	Is a list maintained by the FDA of all drugs manufactured, prepared, propagated, compounded, or processed for commercial distribution
Logical Observation Identifiers Names and Codes	Is a database and universal standard for electronic exchange and gathering of clinical results (such as laboratory tests, clinical observations, outcomes management, and research)
RxNORM	Standardized nomenclature for clinical drugs and drug delivery devices. It links its names to many of the drug vocabularies commonly used in pharmacy management. Maintained by the US National Library of Medicine

APM for Tele-ICU includes Philips VISICU, InTouch Health Remote, and iMDSoft MetaVision ICU. When selecting a system for APM, Tele-ICU programmers should review these FDA requirements. In that situation, the selection is limited between certified technologies or "home-grown" high-standard system.[18]

Isolated central monitoring stations such as Spacelabs Healthcare Xhibit provide remote centralized monitoring and alarm management for groups of patients. They have a unique technical characteristic (as outlined in **Fig. 1**), 24/7 telepresence support and can be used as part of a Tele-ICU system.

Box 1
Additional resources

Center for Connected Health Policy (https://www.cchpca.org) is a nonprofit, nonpartisan organization working to maximize telehealth's ability to improve health outcomes, care delivery, and cost-effectiveness.

Office for the Advancement of Telehealth, Health Resources and Services Administration (OAT/HRSAc; https://www.hrsa.gov/rural-health/telehealth/) promotes the use of telehealth technologies for health care delivery, education, and health information services.

TELEHEALTH Start-Up and Resource Guide (https://www.healthit.gov/sites/default/files/telehealthguide_final_0.pdf; October 2014) created in partnership between Telligen and gpTRAC, the Great Plains Telehealth Resource and Assistance Center.

The Federal Telehealth Compendium (https://www.healthit.gov/sites/default/files/federal_telehealth_compendium_final_122316.pdf; November 2016) contains telehealth activities and resources available across the federal arena.

American Telemedicine Association (http://www.americantelemed.org) ATA is a nonprofit association with a membership network of more than 10,000 industry leaders, and health care professionals entirely focused on telehealth.

Modern providers of telemedicine systems such as Vidyo[19] use technologies that run on windows x-86-compatible servers and multiplatform software that does not require proprietary networking hardware. This is different from most proprietary solutions, such as those offered by Cisco Systems or Polycom.

Classic Tele-ICU allows clinicians to remotely see patients, see bedside monitors, review the patient's past medical history, care plan, test results, and medications. Integrated video/high-quality audio links enable the remote clinician, in real-time, to interact with the patient, bedside nurse, clinician, and the patient's family. This video capability allows the clinician to observe a patient's physical condition and the room. Successful Tele-ICU services support the collaborative care model and remote hospital workflows.

TECHNOLOGY IS IMPORTANT, BUT IT IS NOT EVERYTHING

Tele-ICU programs require technology-enabled data access and communication tools, but success is primarily based on human and organizational factors. Recent clinical and economic evaluation of Tele-ICU shows that, notwithstanding the substantial costs, Tele-ICU programs may reduce ICU and hospital mortality and shorten the length of stay in the ICU,[20] especially when integrated tightly with the bedside care delivery system (**Box 1**).

REFERENCES

1. Telehealth. Available at: https://healthit.ahrq.gov/key-topics/telehealth. Accessed March 31, 2019.
2. Telemedicine Glossary. Available at: https://thesource.americantelemed.org/resources/telemedicine-glossary. Accessed March 31, 2019.
3. Margolis SA, Ypinazar VA. Tele-pharmacy in remote medical practice: the Royal Flying Doctor Service Medical Chest Program. Rural Remote Health 2008;8(2):937.
4. Nicogossian AE, Doarn CR. Armenia 1988 earthquake and telemedicine: lessons learned and forgotten. Telemed J E Health 2011;17(9):741–5.

5. Grundy BL, Crawford P, Jones PK, et al. Telemedicine in critical care: an experiment in health care delivery. JACEP 1977;6(10):439–44.
6. Grundy BL, Jones PK, Lovitt A. Telemedicine in critical care: problems in design, implementation, and assessment. Crit Care Med 1982;10(7):471–5.
7. Rosenfeld BA, Dorman T, Breslow MJ, et al. Intensive care unit telemedicine: alternate paradigm for providing continuous intensivist care. Crit Care Med 2000; 28(12):3925–31.
8. Breslow MJ, Rosenfeld BA, Doerfler M, et al. Effect of a multiple-site intensive care unit telemedicine program on clinical and economic outcomes: an alternative paradigm for intensivist staffing. Crit Care Med 2004;32(1):31–8.
9. Kahn JM, Cicero BD, Wallace DJ, et al. Adoption of ICU telemedicine in the United States. Crit Care Med 2014;42(2):362–8.
10. Kumar S, Merchant S, Reynolds R. Tele-ICU: efficacy and cost-effectiveness approach of remotely managing the critical care. Open Med Inform J 2013;7: 24–9.
11. Celi LA, Hassan E, Marquardt C, et al. The eICU: it's not just telemedicine. Crit Care Med 2001;29(8 Suppl):N183–9.
12. Whitten P, Sypher BD. Evolution of telemedicine from an applied communication perspective in the United States. Telemed J E Health 2006;12(5):590–600.
13. Majerowicz A, Tracy S. Telemedicine: bridging gaps in healthcare delivery. J AHIMA 2010;81(5):52–3, 56.
14. HIPAA Security Rule Standards. Available at: https://hipaaacademy.net/hipaa-security-rule/. Accessed March 31, 2019.
15. eICU program. Telehealth for the intensive care unit. Available at: https://www.usa.philips.com/healthcare/product/HC865325ICU/eicu-program-telehealth-for-the-intensive-care-unit. Accessed March 31, 2019.
16. Code of Federal Regulations 21 Part 880. Docket No. FDA-2008-N-0106. 2008. Available at: https://www.accessdata.fda.gov/scripts/cdrh/cfdocs/cfcfr/CFRSearch.cfm?CFRPart=880. Accessed March 31, 2019.
17. Medical Devices; Medical Device Data Systems. FDA rule 76 FR 8637 , FDA-2008-N-0106. Available at: https://www.federalregister.gov/documents/2011/02/15/2011-3321/medical-devices-medical-device-data-systems. Accessed March 31, 2019.
18. Reynolds HN, Bander J, McCarthy M. Different systems and formats for tele-ICU coverage: designing a tele-ICU system to optimize functionality and investment. Crit Care Nurs Q 2012;35(4):364–77.
19. Personalized Healthcare Without Borders. Available at: https://www.vidyo.com/video-conferencing-solutions/healthcare. Accessed March 31, 2019.
20. Chen J, Sun D, Yang W, et al. Clinical and economic outcomes of telemedicine programs in the intensive care unit: a systematic review and meta-analysis. J Intensive Care Med 2018;33(7):383–93.

Impact of Intensive Care Unit Telemedicine on Outcomes

Isabelle C. Kopec, MD[a,b,*]

KEYWORDS

- ICU telemedicine Outcomes • Tele-ICU results • Telemedicine mortality
- Length of stay • Best practices • ICU telemedicine Implementation
- Telemedicine effectiveness • Telemedicine process of care

KEY POINTS

- The intensivist-led continuous model of intensive care unit (ICU) telemedicine was developed to leverage scarce intensivists and critical care nurses to manage a larger population of patients.
- This ICU telemedicine model has a proven impact on lowering mortality, decreasing length of stay, and improving compliance with best practices.
- The model reviewed is a complex, multimodal reengineering of care delivery. It overlays intensivist patient care, supplemental monitoring and best practice compliance processes, and ICU-specific performance data on existing ICU staff, structures, and processes.
- The effective integration of the ICU telemedicine team with the existing bedside staff and workflows is critical to a successful program. These are explored in this article.
- A successful comprehensive ICU telemedicine program may have other impacts on hospitals and their communities by affecting transfers, centralizing hospital system functions, supporting high acuity areas outside of the ICU, and decreasing burnout of bedside intensivists.

The body of literature on the outcomes of implementing intensive care unit (ICU) telemedicine programs has grown in the past 18 years and is the focus of this review. The initial focus was the impact on mortality and length of stay (LOS) with more recent studies evaluating other factors that contribute to successful results.

Among all models of providing ICU telemedicine, only the predominant model has yielded significant published outcomes data. This model entails continuous monitoring by a remote intensivist-led critical care team, continuous data feeds from the

Disclosure Statement: Co-founder and shareholder, Advanced ICU Care, independent, privately owned acute care telemedicine company.
[a] Advanced ICU Care, One City Place Drive, Suite 570, St Louis, MO 63141, USA; [b] Department of Critical Care Medicine, SSM DePaul, 123030 DePaul Drive, Bridgeton, MO 63044, USA
* Advanced ICU Care, One City Place Drive, Suite 570, St Louis, MO 63141
E-mail address: Isabelle.Kopec@advancedicucare.com

bedside to the remote team, decision support algorithms, real-time alerts, 2-way video communication, population management tools, and reporting solutions.

The first study evaluating the feasibility of leveraging intensivists and critical care nurses through telemedicine was reported by Rosenfeld and colleagues[1] in 2000. They reported a decline in severity-adjusted ICU mortality of 45% and hospital mortality of 30% in one ICU. Breslow and colleagues[2] subsequently described reduced hospital mortality of ICU patients within the post-ICU telemedicine period as well (9.4% vs 12.9%; relative risk [RR] 0.73; 95% confidence interval [CI]0.55–0.95) and shorter ICU LOS (3.63 days: 95% CI 3.21–4.04 vs 4.35 days; 95% CI 3.93–4.78). Breslow and Rosenfeld pioneered this model of intensivist-led continuous care, with population management tools, to leverage critical care providers to cover a larger number of patients over multiple facilities using proprietary software that they developed. It included real-time data feeds, clinical decision support, alerting system, and outcomes and practice metrics.

Other studies followed,[3–9] confirming significant decreases in hospital mortality averaging 20% to 30% and in many cases significantly shorter ICU and/or Hospital LOS for ICU patients (**Table 1**). The ICU telemedicine technology used by McCambridge and colleagues[4] was a different continuous monitoring software but yielded a similar positive impact on mortality.

Over time, however, some hospitals and systems reported a lack of improvement in these global metrics.[10–12] The negative studies brought to light some of the difficulties of implementing an ICU telemedicine program and raised questions about the efficacy of ICU telemedicine.

ICU telemedicine is a different model of critical care, and integrating the ICU telemedicine component with bedside care is complex and changes how critically ill patients are managed. It is *assisted* by technology, but implementing it is a multimodal social and cultural change management initiative with numerous potential points of failure.

There were early indications that the effectiveness of ICU telemedicine systems may be linked to the extent to which the ICU telemedicine intensivists have autonomy to intervene and comanage the patient's care. Those programs with better integration between the bedside and ICU telemedicine teams and more active involvement in patient care by the ICU telemedicine physicians saw positive results.[1–4,6,8,9] Those with little to no improvement in outcomes allowed less involvement by the ICU telemedicine providers.[10,11] Lack of program acceptance and lack of autonomy to treat patients given to the ICU telemedicine team were seen as reasons for program ineffectiveness in impacting mortality or LOS.[10,11]

When early ICU telemedicine programs were implemented, the predominant mode of program implementation gave each bedside physician the option to choose the degree of comanagement "allowed" the ICU telemedicine intensivist. This ranged from "monitor only" (unless the patient is in a life-threatening situation), to "monitor and proceed with standard best practice implementation" to "full comanagement" when the bedside physician was not present.

Nearly 70% of the medical staff in the study by Thomas and colleagues[10] opted out of collaborating with the ICU telemedicine physicians by restricting the intensivist to intervening only in life-threatening situations apparently impacting the results in a negative manner. ICU telemedicine was a new care delivery model and giving bedside physicians the option to "opt out" initially was meant to ease adoption and acceptance by the bedside physicians. It is now well established that high-intensity intensivist involvement is associated with decreased mortality[13] and evidence is growing that active intensivist involvement through ICU telemedicine also contributes to better patient outcomes.[6,14,15]

Table 1
ICU telemedicine outcomes studies

Source	Total Patients	Illness Severity APACHE III/IV Control/ Telemedicine	Key Results
Rosenfeld et al,[1] 2000	628	37/38	30% decrease in hospital mortality, 45% decrease in ICU mortality
Breslow et al,[2] 2004	2140	39/38	RR hospital mortality 0.73 Decrease hospital mortality 9.4% vs 12.9% Decrease ICU LOS 3.63 d vs 4.35 d
Thomas et al,[10] 2009	4142	SAPSII 35/34	No difference in risk-adjusted hospital mortality, RR .85 (95% CI 0.71–1.03), ICU mortality RR .88 (95% CI 0.71–1.08) or LOS. Improved survival in sicker patients
Zawada et al,[3] 2009	2633	38/44	LOS decreased and ICU mortality decreased OR 0.35; $P = .007$. Decreased hospital LOS 10.08 vs 7.81 d; $P = .001$. Decreased ICU LOS 2.08 d vs 3.79 d; $P = .001$
McCambridge et al,[4] 2010	1913	57/58	Hospital mortality decreased by 29%. No change in LOS.
Morrison et al,[11] 2010	4088	49/48	No improvement.
Lilly et al,[6] 2011	6290	45/58	OR 0.40 for hospital mortality, $P = .005$. ICU mortality OR 0.37; $P = .003$ Decrease hospital mortality 11.8% vs 13.6% HR hospital LOS 1.44, $P<.001$, HR ICU LOS 1.26; $P<.001$ Shorter hospital LOS 9.8 d vs 13.3 d. ICU LOS 4.5 d vs 6.4 d
Kohl et al,[32] 2012	1745		A significant decrease in SICU mortality, ICU and hospital LOS vs no decrease in control unit MICU with no telemedicine
Willmitch et al,[8] 2012	24,656	CMI 2.68/2.77	RR of hospital mortality 0.77 $P<.001$ Hospital LOS decreased 14.2%. ICU LOS 12.6% shorter. Hospital LOS lowered to 10.6 d vs 11.86 d; $P<.001$ ICU LOS lowered to 3.80 d vs 4.35 d; $P<.001$

(continued on next page)

Table 1 (continued)			
Source	Total Patients	Illness Severity APACHE III/IV Control/ Telemedicine	Key Results
Lilly et al,[9] 2014	118,990	47/53	HR for hospital mortality 0.84; $P<.001$; ICU mortality HR 0.74; $P<.001$ Decrease in hospital mortality 10% vs 11% Hospital LOS 15% shorter, ICU LOS 20% shorter
Nassar et al,[12] 2014	3355		No significant decrease in ICU, hospital, 30-d mortality or LOS
Fortis et al,[7] 2014	34,406 patient days		25% decrease in mortality Decrease ICU mortality 4.9% vs 6.5%; $P<.0002$

Abbreviations: APACHE, Acute Physiology and Chronic Health Evaluation; CMI, case mix index; HR, hazard risk; ICU, intensive care unit; LOS, length of stay; MICU, medical ICU; OR, odds ratio; RR, relative risk; SAPS, Simplified Acute Physiology Score; SICU, surgical ICU.

In the study by Willmitch and colleagues study[8] of nearly 25,000 patients in 10 ICUs in 5 community hospitals, physicians were assigned to best practice implementations as a default to "nudge"[16] them to what is good for the patient. However, they could choose 1 of the other 2 options: only life-threatening involvement or full comanagement. Ninety-seven percent of physicians remained within the "best practices" whereas only 2% of the providers chose a full partnership. Despite this, the best practices partnership model led to significantly decreased ICU and hospital LOS. The decreases in the hospital mortality, however, were statistically significant only in years 2 and 3 after implementation, not in the first year of the program. It is unclear whether more physicians chose fuller collaboration with the ICU telemedicine intensivist as the program matured, or if trust and better integration evolved. This study brought to light the fact that successful implementation of this complex reengineering of critical care delivery may take time to mature and show results. There is a learning curve for the bedside team as well as the ICU telemedicine team.

META-ANALYSIS

Young and colleagues[17] and Wilcox and Adhikari[18] published meta-analyses on the impact of ICU telemedicine programs on ICU and hospital mortalities and LOS. Young and colleagues[17] searched databases from 1950 through September 2010 and included unpublished data, conference presentations, and abstracts. For the final analysis, 7 published articles and 6 conference abstracts were included covering 35 ICUs and 41,374 patients. The ICU telemedicine intervention included heterogeneous models of care with any telecommunication system, including consulting an intensivist by phone. Their control group consisted of similar ICUs with no telemedicine.

Compared with hospitals without ICU telemedicine, there was a 20% lower mortality in ICUs with telemedicine (odds ratio [OR] 0.80; 95% CI, 0.66–0.97; $P = .02$). There was no significant decrease in hospital mortality (OR 0.82; 95% CI, 0.65–1.03). ICU LOS shortened significantly, with a mean reduction of 1.26 (95% CI, 2.21–0.31) days but the hospital LOS (reduction of 0.64 days) was not significant. Studies were deemed to be of moderate quality. In contrast to all pooled studies, the subset of 5 high-quality studies reviewed by Young and colleagues[17] did show a significant decline in hospital mortality as well with OR 0.74 (95% CI, 0.60–0.92).

The meta-analysis of Wilcox and Adhikari[18] reviewed studies through April of 2012. They were before-after observational studies, with a population just under 48,000 patients in 9 studies. The use of telemedicine was consistently associated with reduced ICU (RR 0.79; 95% CI, 0.65–0.96; $P = .02$) and hospital mortality (RR, 0.83; 95% CI, 0.73–0.94; $P = .004$). Decreases in ICU LOS by 0.62 days (95% CI, 1.21–0.04) and hospital LOS of 1.26 days (95% CI, 2.49–0.03) also were both statistically significant.

A high degree of variability between studies was noted in both meta-analyses with striking heterogeneity of approach to the ICU telemedicine intervention itself.

ICU telemedicine is a complex multimodal intervention that leads to a new culture of treating ICU patients, with an expanded critical care team, and different processes of care.

In 2011, an interdisciplinary working group with members of the Critical Care Societies Collaborative, funded by the Agency for Health Research and Quality, published a paper[19] identifying a broad range of needed research in ICU telemedicine to answer further questions on this model of critical care delivery. The need to better understand organizational readiness, optimal change management practices as they apply to ICU telemedicine, organizational structures of the ICU, and tele-ICU and clinical and operational workflow processes that lead to positive results were cited.[19]

PROCESS OF CARE OUTCOMES

Focus has recently increased on elucidating optimal ICU telemedicine processes of care that impact overall outcomes and influence mortality and LOS. The first study to quantify the impact of ICU telemedicine on best practice adherence was published by Lilly and colleagues.[6] It was a prospective, stepped-wedge clinical practice study of more than 6000 adults admitted to any of 7 ICUs (medical/surgical/cardiovascular) on 2 campuses of an academic medical center with bedside intensivist staffing, multidisciplinary rounds, best practice checklists, and a focus on quality.

In addition to significant decreases in hospital mortality (OR 0.40; 95% CI, 0.31–0.52) and shorter hospital LOS (hazard ratio [HR] for discharge 1.44; 95% CI, 1.33–1.56), the ICU telemedicine intervention period, compared with preintervention was associated with higher rates of best practice adherence for prevention of deep venous thrombosis 99% versus 85%, respectively, OR 15.4 (95% CI, 11.3–21.1), and prevention of stress ulcers 96% versus 83%, OR 4.57 (95% CI, 3.91–5.77); cardiovascular protection 99% versus 80%, OR 30.7 (95% CI, 19.3–49.2); prevention of ventilator-associated pneumonia 52% versus 33%, OR 2.20 (95% CI, 1.79–2.70), lower rates of preventable complications 1.6% versus 13% for ventilator-associated pneumonia, OR, 0.15 (95% CI, 0.09–0.23) and 0.6% versus 1.0% for central catheter–related bloodstream infection, OR 0.50 (95% CI, 0.27–0.93).

Additional insights were gained into the impact on patients admitted at night (8 PM to 8 AM) compared with those admitted during the day (8 AM to 8 PM). Subgroup analysis showed the telemedicine intervention had a greater effect on hospital mortality for patients admitted at night (OR 0.33; CI, 0.18–0.59; $P<.001$) than those who were admitted during the day (OR 0.79; 95% CI, 0.39–1.58). Duration of mechanical ventilation was significantly longer in the preintervention group for those admitted at night (10.2 days; 95% CI, 9.16–11.24) than those admitted during the day (6.9 days; 95% CI, 6.34–7.46; $P<.01$). After the institution of telemedicine, ventilator days for admissions at night compared with during the day were not significantly different (5.8 days vs 5.5 days).

This study[6] demonstrated that adding the ICU telemedicine auditing tools and work-flows to already approved best practices that were tracked with checklists and previous education had a material incremental impact.

ASSOCIATION OF INTENSIVE CARE UNIT AND INTENSIVE CARE UNIT TELEMEDICINE INTEGRATION WITH RESULTS

The question of what factors differentiate ICU telemedicine programs with improvements in mortality, LOS, and the process of care outcomes from those with no improvements continues to be an area of study.

Lilly and colleagues[9] reported a multi-ICU and multisystem study (nearly 120,000 patients in 56 ICUs, 32 hospitals, 19 health care systems) with analysis of the components of the ICU telemedicine intervention that were associated with a decrease in mortality, LOS, or both. Data were used from the eResearch Institute Database, a centralized database of participating ICU telemedicine programs that use the continuous model of ICU telemedicine with Phillips software support. The American College of Chest Physicians ICU Telemedicine Survey instrument was used to survey ICU telemedicine practices.[20]

The following practices were associated with lower mortality, reduced LOS, or both:

a. Earlier involvement of an intensive care specialist (case review within 1 hour of admission to ICU)
b. Timely use of performance data (collected by the ICU telemedicine program), reviewed and acted on by an effective ICU governance team and hospital leadership
c. Higher adherence to ICU best practices
d. Quicker alert responsiveness

In 2016, Hawkins and colleagues[14] published their investigation on the impact of the degree of involvement by the ICU telemedicine providers on LOS. This retrospective, comparative, quantitative analysis was done in 8 medical-surgical ICUs from a single health care system with high-intensity intensivist staffing, standard protocols for common ICU problems, and a culture of promoting high levels of adherence to the ICU best practices.

The well-integrated telemedicine ICUs with full comanagement authority methods were associated with significantly shorter ICU and hospital LOS and a higher number of ICU telemedicine orders. This comanagement method was termed the "direct intervention with timely notification" strategy. Acuity-adjusted hospital LOS was significantly lower for "direct intervention with timely notification" comanagement strategy (0.68; 0.65–0.70) compared with a mixed methods group (0.70; 0.69–0.72; $P = .01$), which was in turn significantly lower than a "monitor and notify" group (0.83; 0.80–0.86; $P<.001$). Likewise, fully integrated units had a significantly larger proportion of provider orders recorded by ICU telemedicine physicians than the mixed methods of comanagement groups, which in turn had a larger proportion than ICUs that used the "monitor and notify method" ($P<.001$).

The ICUs supported by the ICU telemedicine program were either staffed with bedside intensivists 24 hours a day and 7 days a week or 12 hours a day and 7 days a week. The ICUs with 24 hours a day bedside intensivists chose the least active role for the ICU telemedicine program and had the longest LOS.

The research agenda in the ICU telemedicine workgroup called for better tools and a better understanding of the links between ICU processes and outcomes.[19] Kahn and colleagues[15] published an ethnographic study analyzing differences in structure, process, implementation, and leadership between ICU telemedicine hospitals that have decreased mortality and/or LOS and those that have no observed change or worse outcomes after implementing ICU telemedicine. They found that the effectiveness in the continuous monitoring and 24/7 model of ICU telemedicine is significantly influenced by the interaction of factors within 3 key domains: leadership of both target ICU and the facility providing remote care, the perceived value of telemedicine by frontline care providers, and the organizational characteristics of the hospital and ICU telemedicine program.

Within each of these domains, key areas of focus requiring optimal implementation emerged. In the leadership domain, decisions on the role of the telemedicine team, conflict resolution, and relationship building were critical factors. Perceived value domain expectations of availability and impact of the program, staff satisfaction, and understanding of operations differentiated programs with positive outcomes. In the organizational characteristics domain, staffing models allowed the involvement of the telemedicine unit/protocols for engagement, and new-hire orientation were key factors. The investigators restricted the study to programs that provided continuous ICU telemedicine services from a centralized location, as this is the predominant model.[20]

Insights from the theory of organizational readiness for change and the role of management in preparing organizations to implement a new process were used in another study.[21] The investigators noted the importance of the ICU telemedicine program to deliver on all components of the multifaceted program (monitoring, evidence-based practices, adding expertise, collecting and utilizing performance data) responsively, consistently, and in a well-integrated manner with the bedside team. Forming 1 care team, with each member understanding their roles and responsibilities and each actively contributing to the patient's care, led to improvements in mortality. In contrast, in sites without decreases in mortality after adoption, the bedside and ICU telemedicine groups remained separate, and the telemedicine staff were often relegated to "observer" status.

In looking at protocols of engagement of the ICU telemedicine critical care team, the degree of autonomy granted the ICU telemedicine team reflects the degree of integration and impacts success.

HOSPITAL IMPACTS

The literature on the impact of ICU telemedicine on hospitals, hospital systems, and health care policy implications is in its early stages. A New England Healthcare Institute (NEHI) demonstration project[5] evaluated the potential impact of an effectively implemented ICU telemedicine program if implemented statewide. In addition to 350 additional lives saved annually in Massachusetts, the effects of the shorter LOS on ICU bed availability, case volume, and throughput, positively impacted hospitals. The savings to payors were estimated to exceed $122 million dollars annually.[5] The financial impact and broader health care impacts are covered later in this article.

Changes in hospital processes, ICU utilization, and acceleration of adoption of best practices, which result from effective ICU-ICU telemedicine performance data review have not been quantified. This is in part because the goals of implementing the program, and whether they were achieved, as well as the specifics of the ICU telemedicine intervention, have not been well characterized in most studies.

ICU telemedicine provides a broader geographic distribution and availability of intensivist expertise so that more patients can be safely managed at community hospitals, while also supporting bedside intensivists wherever they practice. ICU tele-medicine may shift patients to receive care at their local community hospitals, to the extent that local resources allow, reserving transfers to tertiary and quaternary centers for more specialized expertise or interventions. The NEHI report[5] concluded that ICU telemedicine enabled community hospitals to keep more patients, at a lower cost of care than transferring them to tertiary centers.

One recent study found fewer transfers to higher levels of care, with no deleterious effect on mortality,[22] whereas another[23] showed an increase in transfers within the system with no effect on mortality. In the latter study, the observed increase in inter-hospital transfers to their quaternary center after institution of ICU telemedicine ($P = .040$) was seen to a greater extent from less resourced/specialized ICUs ($P = .037$) in comparison with more resourced centers ($P = .88$). This is while Fortis and colleagues[22] compared patient transfers from ICU telemedicine–supported ICUs (52 ICUs in 23 acute care facilities) with transfers from ICUs without ICU telemed-icine support (254 ICUs in 94 facilities). Transfers decreased significantly (from 3.46% to 1.99%) in telemedicine-supported hospitals compared with those in non-telemedicine facilities (2.03% to 1.68%), between pre-ICU and post-ICU telemedicine implementation periods ($P<.001$). After adjusting for demographics, illness severity, diagnosis, and facility, ICU telemedicine was associated with overall reduced transfers with an RR of 0.79 (95% CI, 0.71–0.87; $P<.001$). This reduction was seen with moder-ate (RR 0.77), moderate to high (RR 0.79), and high illness severity (RR 0.73; 95% CI, 0.60–0.90; $P = .003$). Patients with gastrointestinal (RR 0.55, $P<.001$) and respiratory diagnoses (RR 0.52 $P<.001$) had the most significant decreases in transfers.

There was no increase in 30-day mortality in the telemedicine-supported hospitals. More information is needed to assess whether transfers occur strictly for services not provided. As with all aspects of ICU telemedicine implementation, managing trans-fers to a higher level of care requires active management and leadership in many of the same domains as program implementation such as clear goals, buy-in from frontline providers, collaboration, mutually agreed on guidelines, understanding of the ICU telemedicine operations, and ability to support patients who were historically transferred. The ICU telemedicine providers need to be aware of service limitations at the hospital.

Expansion of and support of other service lines within a hospital and improving ICU utilization based on ICU telemedicine data have not been quantified. ICU telemedicine centers are expanding their functions in some cases, to include system level triage, centralized pharmacy oversight,[24] nutrition support services.[25]

Some ICU telemedicine programs have extended the involvement of the ICU tele-medicine team to other high acuity areas, such as Emergency Departments, Post Anesthesia Care Unit and the Progressive Care Unit (PCU). Armaignac and col-leagues[26] found a 20% survival benefit for PCUs with telemedicine support. While the mean PCU LOS was lower (2.6 vs 3.2 days; $P<.001$), the post-PCU hospital LOS was longer for the telemedicine PCU group (7.3 vs 6.8 days; $P<.0001$).

PATIENTS AND PROVIDERS

Patient-specific impacts such as functional status and discharge site have not been studied broadly. One successfully implemented telemedicine program[6] noted more discharges to home after the ICU telemedicine intervention (53.4% after vs 45.9% before, $P<.001$). The effects of ICU telemedicine programs on quality of life, retention, and longevity of bedside intensivists and critical care nurses has not been investigated nor has the impact of the presence of ICU telemedicine support in intensivists' job seeking decisions and recruitment. However, this could potentially play a substantial role with the ongoing shortage of intensivists.

ICU telemedicine has been well accepted by residents[27–29] and is perceived as having a positive effect on their education and support, but some loss of autonomy and decrease in confidence in independently caring for critically ill patients has been noted and needs further quantitative evaluation. The lack of published data in these areas are due in part to the fact that these components of the full ICU telemedicine intervention are not always applicable to all hospitals, and the intervention itself is variably applied.[15,20] Until recently, research has focused primarily on mortality and LOS endpoints. As we gain more experience with ICU telemedicine, we need to refine our knowledge to focus on optimal environments, leadership, and clinical and organizational practices.

Further studies may enhance our knowledge on which patients and ICU structures will benefit most from ICU telemedicine, once we have a more consistent process for successfully implementing this complex, multifaceted intervention. With time, there will be more data to evaluate process, mortality and LOS outcomes on the consultative and/or rounding model that utilizes the intensivist consultation model of ICU telemedicine. Currently, the published data with this model of ICU telemedicine has been primarily in tele-neurology[30] and pediatric patients.[31]

FINAL THOUGHTS

Our understanding of how to optimally use ICU telemedicine to improve clinical care is significantly improved but still evolving. To date, our learnings as a medical community have acknowledged the complexity of a comprehensive ICU telemedicine intervention with multiple codependent components that all need to be effectively implemented to be successful. This is not purely a technological advancement. It is a change in culture and reengineering of the processes of managing ICU patients needed to distribute critical care expertise more broadly and to use the bedside intensivists optimally. The broader impact on the delivery of intensivist expertise, impact on costs of care, the health of communities and hospital to home status will drive future health care policy.

REFERENCES

1. Rosenfeld BA, Dorman T, Breslow MJ, et al. Intensive care unit telemedicine: alternate paradigm for providing continuous intensivist care. Crit Care Med 2000;28:3925–31.
2. Breslow MJ, Rosenfeld BA, Doerfler M, et al. Effect of a multiple-site intensive care unit telemedicine program on clinical and economic outcomes: an alternative paradigm for intensivist staffing. Crit Care Med 2004;32:31–8.
3. Zawada ET Jr, Herr P, Larson D, et al. Impact of an intensive care unit telemedicine program on a rural health care system. Postgrad Med 2009;121:160–70.
4. McCambridge M, Jones K, Paxton H, et al. Association of health information technology and teleintensivist coverage with decreased mortality and ventilator use in critically ill patients. Arch Intern Med 2010;170:648–53.
5. Fifer S, Everett W, Adams M, et al. Critical care, critical choices: the case for tele-ICUs in intensive care. Cambridge (MA): Massachusetts Technology Collaborative; New England Healthcare Institute; 2010.
6. Lilly CM, Cody S, Zhao H, et al. Hospital mortality, length of stay, and preventable complications among critically ill patients before and after tele-ICU reengineering of critical care processes. JAMA 2011;305:2175–83.

7. Fortis S, Weinert C, Bushinski R, et al. A health system-based critical care program with a novel tele-ICU: implementation, cost, and structure details. J Am Coll Surg 2014;219:676–83.

8. Willmitch B, Golembeski S, Kim SS, et al. Clinical outcomes after telemedicine intensive care unit implementation. Crit Care Med 2012;40:450–4.

9. Lilly CM, McLaughlin JM, Zhao H, et al. A multicenter study of ICU telemedicine reengineering of adult critical care. Chest 2014;145:500–7.

10. Thomas EJ, Lucke JF, Wueste L, et al. Association of telemedicine for remote monitoring of intensive care patients with mortality, complications, and length of stay. JAMA 2009;302:2671–8.

11. Morrison JL, Cai Q, Davis N, et al. Clinical and economic outcomes of the electronic intensive care unit: results from two community hospitals. Crit Care Med 2010;38:2–8.

12. Nassar BS, Vaughan-Sarrazin MS, Jiang L, et al. Impact of an intensive care unit telemedicine program on patient outcomes in an integrated health care system. JAMA Intern Med 2014;174:1160–7.

13. L. H. S. R. Series. Bibliography: ICU Physician Staffing. Available at: http://www.leapfroggroup.org/sites/default/files/Files/IPSBibliography.pdf. Accessed January 10, 2019.

14. Hawkins HA, Lilly CM, Kaster DA, et al. ICU telemedicine comanagement methods and length of stay. Chest 2016;150:314–9.

15. Kahn JM, Lilly CM, et al. The research agenda in ICU telemedicine: a statement from the Critical Care Societies Collaborative. Chest 2011;140:230–8.

16. Thaler R, Sunstein C. Nudge: improving decisions about health, wealth, and happiness. New Haven (CT): Yale University Press; 2008. Penguin Books; Revised & Expanded edition.

17. Young LB, Chan PS, Cram P. Staff acceptance of tele-ICU coverage: a systematic review. Chest 2011;139:279–88.

18. Wilcox ME, Adhikari NK. The effect of telemedicine in critically ill patients: systematic review and meta-analysis. Crit Care 2012;16:R127.

19. Kahn JM, Rak KJ, Kuza CC, et al. Determinants of intensive care unit telemedicine effectiveness: an ethnographic study. Am J Respir Crit Care Med 2018. https://doi.org/10.1164/rccm.201802-0259OC.

20. Lilly CM, Fisher KA, Ries M, et al. A national ICU telemedicine survey: validation and results. Chest 2012;142:40–7.

21. Weiner BJ. A theory of organizational readiness for change. Implement Sci 2009; 4:67.

22. Fortis S, Sarrazin MV, Beck BF, et al. ICU telemedicine reduces interhospital ICU transfers in the Veterans Health Administration. Chest 2018;154:69–76.

23. Pannu J, Sanghavi D, Sheley T, et al. Impact of telemedicine monitoring of community ICUs on interhospital transfers. Crit Care Med 2017;45:1344–51.

24. Forni A, Skehan N, Hartman CA, et al. Evaluation of the impact of a tele-ICU pharmacist on the management of sedation in critically ill mechanically ventilated patients. Ann Pharmacother 2010;44:432–8.

25. Sriram K, Nikolich S, Ries M. eNutrition: an extension of teleintensive care. Nutrition 2015;31:1165–7.

26. Armaignac DL, Saxena A, Rubens M, et al. Impact of telemedicine on mortality, length of stay, and cost among patients in progressive care units: experience from a large healthcare system. Crit Care Med 2018;46:728–35.

27. Coletti C, Elliott DJ, Zubrow MT. Resident perceptions of a tele-intensive care unit implementation. Telemed J E Health 2010;16:894–7.

28. Romig MC, Latif A, Gill RS, et al. Perceived benefit of a telemedicine consultative service in a highly staffed intensive care unit. J Crit Care 2012;27:426.e9-16.
29. Summe A, Foor L, Hoeck L, et al. Resident perceptions of competency and comfort before and after telemedicine-ICU implementation. South Med J 2018;111: 344-7.
30. Vespa PM, Miller C, Hu X, et al. Intensive care unit robotic telepresence facilitates rapid physician response to unstable patients and decreased cost in neurointensive care. Surg Neurol 2007;67:331-7.
31. Marcin JP, Nesbitt TS, Kallas HJ, et al. Use of telemedicine to provide pediatric critical care inpatient consultations to underserved rural Northern California. J Pediatr 2004;144:375-80.
32. Kohl BA, Fortino-Mullen M, Praestgaard A, et al. The effect of ICU telemedicine on mortality and length of stay. J Telemed Telecare 2012;18:282-6.

Quality Improvement and Telemedicine Intensive Care Unit: A Perfect Match

Devang K. Sanghavi, MBBS, MD[a], Pramod K. Guru, MBBS, MD[a],
Pablo Moreno Franco, MD[b],*

KEYWORDS

• Critical care • Quality improvement • Tele-ICU • Communication

KEY POINTS

• Telemedicine intensive care can potentially participate in the care of critically ill patients by covering hospital in a multitude of ways.

• The eventual care and overall improvement in the quality of care provided by the telemedicine intensive care team depends on the teams' composition and its relationship with the local practice.

• We describe the synergistic role that quality improvement methodology plays to assist with both implementation science and to facilitate a successful collaboration between the local intensive care practice and the telemedicine team.

INTRODUCTION

There are approximately 5980 intensive care units (ICUs) in the United States caring for about 55,000 patients a day. Based on the results of a survey published by Angus and colleagues,[1] only 4% of the ICU had dedicated attending daytime coverage and any evening physician coverage. Fifty percent of the ICUs had no intensivist coverage, 20% had weekday coverage, 12% had weeknight coverage, and 10% had weekend day coverage, presenting a substantial need for telemedicine intensive care teams (Tele-ICU).

Tele-ICU was first showcased in 1977 as a tool with the potential to enhance care for patients in a smaller private hospital monitored from an academic medical center.[2] Tele-ICU adoption increased from 16 hospitals and 598 beds in 2002 to 213 hospitals and 5799 beds in 2010, based on data from the Centers for Medicare and Medicaid

Conflict of Interest: None.
[a] Department of Critical Care Medicine, Mayo Clinic, 4500 San Pablo Road, Jacksonville, FL 32224, USA; [b] Division of Transplant Medicine, Department of Critical Care Medicine, Mayo Clinic, 4500 San Pablo Road, Jacksonville, FL 32224, USA
* Corresponding author.
E-mail address: MorenoFranco.Pablo@mayo.edu

Crit Care Clin 35 (2019) 451–462
https://doi.org/10.1016/j.ccc.2019.02.003
0749-0704/19/© 2019 Elsevier Inc. All rights reserved.

Services.[3] Tele-ICU programs support 11% of nonfederal hospital critically ill patients.[4] This number is only going to increase as the quantity of practicing intensivists remain stagnant and demand for around-the-clock specialized intensivist care continues to increase nationwide.[5] The intensivist supply–demand gap seems to be even more marked in rural areas, so the availability of Tele-ICU services guarantees that, in a timely manner, trained specialists are able to assess patients and guide therapy. Without Tele-ICU, patients either have to be transferred to higher levels of care or forgo specialty care; in both of these cases, a margin for error increases and unnecessary delays in care may be introduced.

Beyond increased availability and enhanced timeliness of care, other substantial advantages that Tele-ICU coverage can provide are standardization and continuity of care. The scope of involvement of the Tele-ICU physician can be further classified into comanagement, consultation, and emergent care. The eventual care and the overall improvement in the quality of care provided by the Tele-ICU depend on the composition of the Tele-ICU team, which can potentially include physicians, Advanced Practice Providers (APP), and nurses.[6] The Tele-ICU center can be staffed within the system, wherein the hospital system can manage the Tele-ICU with their clinicians and nurses or outsource it to a vendor that operates a network of ICUs.[2]

There are risks and opportunities that arise as the tele-ICU model is incorporated to an existing local ICU practice, because of the potential differences in policies, procedures, protocols, and process and outcome metrics, along with variations in clinical practice. Potential miscommunication could lead to significant problems in providing appropriate care. That being said, when the tele-ICU implementation process is complete, using quality improvement (QI) methodology, there are many potential advantages. For example, QI has a proven record of closing the gap between evidence-based medicine and clinical practice, bringing the framework and tools that support the implementation of best practices while tracking meaningful outcome indicators and relevant process metrics.

MEDICAL ERRORS IN THE INTENSIVE CARE UNIT AND INCREASING SAFETY IN TELE-INTENSIVE CARE USING QUALITY IMPROVEMENT TOOLS

According to reports from the Agency for Healthcare Research and Quality, roughly 10% of ICU patients develop an adverse effect such as a health care-associated infection, pressure ulcer, preventive all medication-related event, or a fall during hospitalization.[7] Some other potential complications associated with ICU care have frequently been described in the literature and include deep vein thrombosis, pulmonary embolism, gastrointestinal bleeding, catheter-associated urinary tract infection, central line-associated bloodstream infections, ventilator-associated pneumonia, delirium, and acute lung injury.

One of the most critical elements in any industry is QI. The safety level required in each industry determines the extent of the resources needed to achieve it. QI can assist to find a balance between achieving an appropriate level of safety with the correct amount of resources. The spectrum of expected safety could go from ultrasafe industries (eg, commercial aviation; processing industries), which refers to those industries in which safety and the means to achieve it are the absolute priority to ultra-adaptive industries (eg, combat flight, Himalaya mountaineering) that rely heavily on each individuals judgment, adaptability, and resilience, and finally the high-reliability industries (eg, chartered flights), which implies that the teams exhibit characteristics that allow them to operate both in safe conditions and flexibility to respond and manage risk.[8] In medicine, a similar spectrum can be conceived, going from avoiding risk in ultrasafe radiation therapy, managing risk in highly reliable anesthesiology, and mitigating adverse events in ultraadaptive trauma surgery. As in ICUs, clinical providers need to include safety, high reliability, and adaptability moving from ultrasafe conditions to ultraadaptive conditions in emergency situations; therefore, the use of QI in ICUs gains even more relevance to ensure safety.

QUALITY IMPROVEMENT METHODOLOGY EXAMPLES: PLAN–DO–STUDY–ACT CYCLES, DEFINE–MEASURE–ANALYZE–IMPROVE–CONTROL, AND LEAN
Cause and Effect Diagram

Cause and effect diagrams are visual tools designed to group steps and enumerate them in the logical order of the substeps within a process that could breakdown to produce a failure or defect. Very commonly, fishbone diagrams are used to represent causes and effects.

Driver Diagram

Once we understand that each process has steps that are critical to quality and that the visual depiction in a driver diagram helps to identify risks of each stage. Then, attention can be turned to further mitigate the risks based on the primary and secondary drivers. Each one of these drivers could influence performance to a certain degree.

Define–Measure–Analyze–Improve–Control

Define–Measure–Analyze–Improve–Control is one of the most comprehensives tools. It describes the 5 required steps to guide QI projects and teams. Each step is further defined in **Fig. 1**. It is important to mention that all of the requirements in each step are completed before moving to the next stage.

Metrics

To make sure every intervention is leading to a better patient-related outcome, appropriate quality metrics should be defined and tracked. Typically, these metrics can be

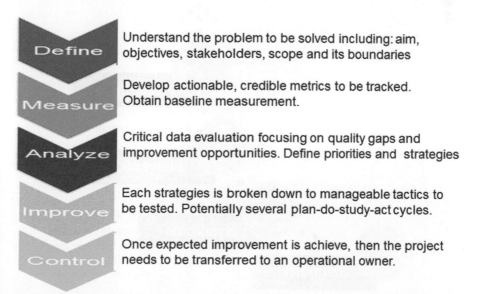

Define — Understand the problem to be solved including: aim, objectives, stakeholders, scope and its boundaries

Measure — Develop actionable, credible metrics to be tracked. Obtain baseline measurement.

Analyze — Critical data evaluation focusing on quality gaps and improvement opportunities. Define priorities and strategies

Improve — Each strategies is broken down to manageable tactics to be tested. Potentially several plan-do-study-act cycles.

Control — Once expected improvement is achieve, then the project needs to be transferred to an operational owner.

Fig. 1. Define–measure–analyze–improve–control: the 5 phases of the methodology.

divided into 2 groups: process and outcome. The health care delivery process ultimately is focused on delivering safety, health maintenance, and patient satisfaction; therefore, outcome metrics should be aligned with patient-related outcomes. When we engineer ICUs, it is recommended that the performance of each critical-to-quality step is tracked as a process metric, which could be done using tele-ICU resources.

Failure Modes and Effects Analysis

Failure modes and effects analysis is one of the most powerful improvement tools, in which all the identified different potential failure modes are stratified in terms of their risk priority index. The frequency, severity, and potential safety mechanisms are accounted for to determine relative importance.

Flowchart

A flowchart is a schematic representation of the different inputs and processes required to deliver high quality to the patient or customers.

Plan–Do–Study–Act Cycles

A plan–do–study–act cycles is a structured approach that uses repeated attempts to modify a process to optimize the performance. Application of consecutive plan–do–study–act cycles in ICU care is essential to improve quality of care (**Fig. 2**).

TELE-INTENSIVE CARE AND ITS ROLE IN ENHANCING INTENSIVE CARE UNIT QUALITY OF CARE

Some of the landmark studies supporting the use of Tele-ICU have been closely linked to specific QI activities. Using QI in Tele-ICU in one study led to an improvement in evidence-based practices adherence and prevention of ICU adverse events.[9]

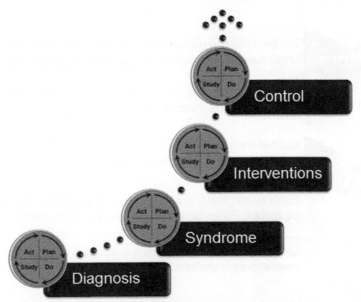

Fig. 2. Plan–do–study–act cycles: a common framework to both critical care and QI.

Providing intensive care requires a fast pace to move from escalation of care to procedures, adaptation, prevention, deescalation, and recovery, which can create tremendous variation in ICU care depending on resources including provider availabilities, ICU census, and patient acuity, among others.

Because of Tele-ICUs advantages in timeliness along with standardization and continuity in care, having a well-organized Tele-ICU team supervising the operation can enhance the safety, patient and provider experience, and quality outcomes. In a systematic review, both centralized monitoring and virtual consultant models have shown improvement in clinical practice adherence.[10]

Length of Stay

Two systematic reviews have been performed to assess the impact of Tele-ICU on patient outcomes, including length of stay. The first by Young and colleagues[11] included 13 eligible studies in 35 ICUs, all of which used a before and after design. The results of this review did not show Tele-ICU coverage to decrease the ICU length of stay (mean difference, −0.64 days; 95% confidence interval [CI], −1.52 to 0.25; P = .16).[11] The second study included 11 articles and reported statistically significant differences in ICU and hospital length of stay (weighted mean difference [telemedicine control], −0.62 days [95% CI −1.21 to −0.04] and −1.26 days [95% CI, −2.49 to −0.03], respectively).[12]

Mortality Impact: Intensive Care Unit and Inpatient

Young and colleagues[11] showed an association between Tele-ICU monitoring and a decrease in ICU mortality (pooled odds ratio [OR], 0.80; 95% CI, 0.66–0.97; P = .02), but not in-hospital mortality for patients admitted to an ICU (pooled OR, 0.82; 95% CI, 0.65–1.03; P = .08). Wilcox and Adhikari[12] Also reported Tele-ICU, compared with standard of care, is associated with a lower ICU (risk ratio, 0.79; 95% CI, 0.65–0.96; 9 studies; n = 23,526 participants) and hospital mortality (risk ratio, 0.83; 95% CI, 0.73–0.94; 9 studies; n = 47,943 participants).

Another systematic review, including only randomized controlled trials and quasiexperimental studies, questioned the methodologic quality of most studies investigating Tele-ICU. This systematic review only included 2 studies meeting the eligibility criteria of appropriate methodology. The first, a nonrandomized, stepped-wedge design in 7 ICUs, showed a decrease in hospital mortality from 13.6% (95% CI, 11.9%–15.4%) to 11.8% (95% CI, 10.9%–12.8%) during the intervention period, with an adjusted OR of 0.40 (95% CI, 0.31–0.52; P = .005).[9] The second study, an unblinded, nonrandomized, preassessment/postassessment of Tele-ICU in 56 adult ICUs, reported a reduction in hospital mortality from 11% to 10% (adjusted hazard ratio, 0.84; 95% CI, 0.78–0.89; P<.001).[13] Both studies confirm a decrease in hospital mortality in patients receiving Tele-ICU care, and they assert that more multisite, randomized, controlled trials or quasiexperimental studies are needed to determine the implementation cost and effectiveness of the intervention.[14]

Intensive Care Unit Emergencies

A significant advantage of Tele-ICU is the ability for alerts and alarms to be initiated by off-site personnel in addition to the standard in-house bedside staff. In a study performed by the University of Massachusetts, most of the day interventions were initiated by the Tele-ICU group.[9] During the Tele-ICU period, there were 6.80 alerts (95% CI, 6.50–7.10) for physiologic instability per patient per day, and from those, 1.75 alerts (95% CI, 1.69–1.81) were managed with a Tele-ICU intervention.[9] The human factor approach and the impact of such alerts in alarm fatigue and staff burnout should be better characterized in future studies.

CONTINUOUS QUALITY IMPROVEMENT BY TELE-INTENSIVE CARE

The concept that every system is perfectly designed to achieve the results has become fashionable in the health care improvement industry. But taking these concepts a little further, one could conceptualize designing a health care system in which every safety event is used as a learning opportunity. Subsequently, QI methodology could be applied to prevent similar events in the future. Then, a continuously learning health care delivery system is born. We propose here that the collaboration between Tele-ICU and local ICU to examine safety events, generate improvement projects, and track metrics will enhance patient outcomes.

LEVERAGING CURRENT AND FUTURE KNOWLEDGE TO ENHANCE INTENSIVE CARE UNIT METRICS BY TELE-INTENSIVE CARE

Many of the diagnostic criteria or risk stratification scoring systems available in the ICU have been the product of traditional research, mainly using logistic regression modeling. One of the limitations of such traditionally derived tools is that only a relatively small number of patients and data points were used to drive them. With the promise of big data, machine learning, and artificial intelligence, one could conceptualize a new future in which Tele-ICU monitoring will also serve as an avenue to capture data, identify variations in care, and follow trends. The data being captured could, in turn, be used to apply machine learning algorithms that can improve the performance of risk stratification models and artificial intelligence–derived decision support tools.

RESOURCE USE AND PROJECT PRIORITIZATION

As the need for appropriate QI projects continues to grow, it is important to identify projects with higher priorities that have more impact and need fewer resources to achieve their goals. Project prioritization is a very simple but very powerful approach that could potentially be used in all ICUs as well as during or after the deployment of a Tele-ICU service. The process steps are as follows.

1. Establish the degree of impact that each QI project will have in the spoke of hub ICU.
2. Define the effort level that will be required, which in part depends on the size of each project.
3. Along with other stakeholders, create an impact–effort prioritization grid or priority matrix.[15]

A frequent question that arises when trying to define the effort that will be required to complete a project is how to determine the scope of the project in a way that could be compared with other projects. **Table 1** proposes a number of elements that could be considered to determine projects scope. **Table 2** demonstrate the calculation of priority score and risk priority matrix. **Table 2** shows how to calculate the impact score by the impact of the project to improve access throughput or clinical outcomes, increase patient safety, enhance public image, improve patient experience and compliance with regulatory requirements, and effects on other stakeholders. **Table 2b** describes the calculation of the estimated effort required for each project. The variables that are taken into account include project scope, extent of time to completion, amount of data needs to be tracked, the data sources including whether or not the

Table 1
Plan-do-study-act cycles: a common framework to both critical care and QI

Characteristics	Small and Just Do It	Medium	Large	Extra-Large
Scope example	Single ICU	2 ICUs	2–5 ICUs	>5 ICUs
Speed to mobilize	Rapid	Rapid	Slow	Very Slow
QI expert	From the local practice	From the practice or Tele-ICU	From other areas of the hospital	From outside company
Duration	Days to weeks	Days to <3 mo	3–6 mo	6–24 mo
Cost	Teeny	Small	Big	Bigger
Control	Pulled in	Pulled in–pushed down	Pulled in–pushed down	Pushed down
Sustainability	Easy	Easy–ok	Hard	Very hard
Diffusion of best practices	Usually not required But easily done	Sometimes required Needs some work	Hard	Very hard, usually not needed
Decision drivers	Close to the process/ patients	Close to the process/ patients	Removed from patient/process	Very removed from patient/ process
Patient/voice of the costumer involvement	Easy	Easy–ok	Hard	Very hard
Change management required	Barely any/ crowd sourcing	Some but limited to those areas no time required	Moderate to large, usually no time required	Moderate to large, may require some time
Data required	Available within Tele-ICU or IT	Requires IT or extra resources from Tele-ICU to pull	Requires IT, Tele-ICU and EHR vendor	Requires IT, Tele-ICU, EHR vendor and outside agency
Impact	Small	Moderate	Large	Huge
Risk	Minimal	Moderate	Large	Huge
RPN (15 areas)	<50	50–75	75–120	>120

Abbreviations: EHR, electronic health records; IT, information technology; RPN, risk priority number.

data already exists or needs to be generated, estimation of the required change management efforts, potential cost, availability of infrastructure and historical assessment regarding similar projects that may have been completed before.

Once the impact and effort scoring of all proposed projects are calculated, an impact–effort risk priority matrix can be built to guide resource use (**Table 2**c).

DIFFUSION OF BEST PRACTICES ACROSS ALL INTENSIVE CARE UNITS

For the success of a health care institution, the adoption and implementation of best practices to the bedside for all patients and consistency in health care delivery across the entire system are necessary. Some of the challenges on the path to success,

Table 2
Impact effort grid for tele-ICU QI projects prioritization

A. Impact scoring

Access to Increase	Outcomes to Improve	Safety to Improve	Public Image to Impact	Patient and Person Experience to Improve	Regulatory Requirement Driven	System/Structure Already in Place	Risk Priority Number
0 N/A	0 N/A	0 N/A	0 N/A	0 N/A	0 Low	0—yes, good	
3 small	3 soft	3 mild	3 mild	3 some	3 Some $	3—borderline	
5 medium	5 medium	5 moderate	5 moderate	5 moderate	5 Moderate $$	5—weak	
10 Strong	10 Important	10 Significant	10 Strong	10 Important	10 High $$$	10—no	

B. Effort scoring

Scope	Speed	Data Required	Resources Required	Change Management Required	Cost	Structure Already in Place?	Similar Project Successfully Completed before?	Risk Priority Number
0 small	0 fast	0 none	0 none	0 none	0 low	0—yes, strong	0—yes, strong	
3 M	3 mid	3 some	3 some	3 some	3 some $	3—moderate	3—moderate	
5 L	5 slow	5 a lot	5 a lot	5 a lot	5 moderate $$	5—weak	5—weak	
10 XL	10 extra slow	10 huge	10 huge	10 huge	10 high $$$	10—no	10—no	

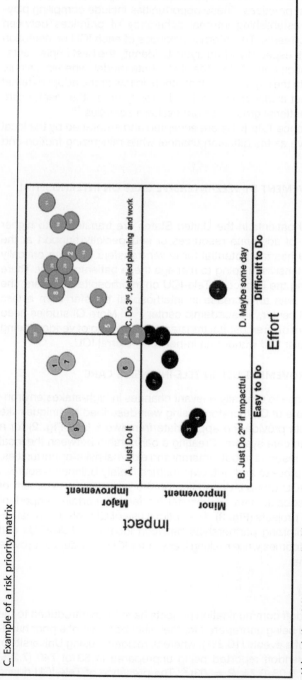

C. Example of a risk priority matrix

Abbreviation: N/A, not applicable.

include identification of appropriate best practices, infrastructure to measure and report data, integration into electronic health record, protected time for providers guiding implementation, competing priorities that could affect the speed of diffusion, and cultural challenges to standardized work.[16]

The Tele-ICU infrastructure provides several potential advantages in both discovery and dissemination on the best practices. These opportunities include compiling playbooks with best practices, establishing internal coherency of practices between different ICUs, and organizing teams. The internal dynamics of each ICU or institution need to be taken into account, especially when trying to identify the best implementation approach. Practice adoption could follow the alpha–beta model, wherein a single site defines best practices with the expectation that others follow or the adopt external practices model, in which best evidence is translated directly from other health care organizations, government, national groups, or professional societies.[16]

The big advantage is that, once Tele-ICUs are accepted and embraced by the local ICU practice, then it can serve as the diffusion channel while minimizing friction and maximizing standardization.

IMPACT OF QUALITY IMPROVEMENT BY TELE-INTENSIVE CARE ON INTERHOSPITAL TRANSFERS

Approximately 5% of all ICU patients in the United States are transferred to higher care level centers for a lack of adequate resources or subspecialty support at the referring hospital.[17] Tele-ICU has the potential for fewer transfers of these critically ill patients with a Tele-ICU intensivist helping to manage these patients locally. There are few publications regarding the impact of Tele-ICU on interhospital transfers; the authors reported that there was an increase in interhospital transfer from a less resourced ICU to the referral center, an academic center.[18,19] More QI studies need to be conducted on the pattern of interhospital transfers in the setting of vendors being contracted to cover a particular ICU without an in-network referral ICU.

CONTINUOUS QUALITY IMPROVEMENT USE IN TELE-INTENSIVE CARE

Improving appropriate response to clinically relevant changes in high-stakes environments like an ICU is at the core of QI; therefore, using well-described techniques like plan–do–study–act cycles can provide the appropriate framework (see **Fig. 2**) for a continuously improving health care system. Creating a partnership between the local ICU practice and Tele-ICU to respond to both internal and external risks/opportunities, aggregating data from both process and outcome metrics, safely balance resources provided by local and Tele-ICU groups, depending on the proactive assessment of the degree of risk, and feedback data to hospital leadership pertains important Tele-ICU related potential QI projects (**Fig. 3**). The optimal use of QI tools when establishing, developing, and optimizing partnerships between local and Tele-ICUs can result in improved patient outcomes while making it easier for ICU providers to provide the right care at the right time.

HANDOFF COMMUNICATION

Even after standardized handoff communication projects have been introduced to the ICU, clinicians have reported being unprepared for their shift because of a poor handoff quality in 35 of 343 handoffs events (10.2%), whereas residents using University of Washington Standardized Handoff reported being unprepared in 53 of 740 (7.2%) handoffs (OR, 0.19; 95% CI, 0.03–0.74; $P = .03$).[20] The presence of Tele-ICU during

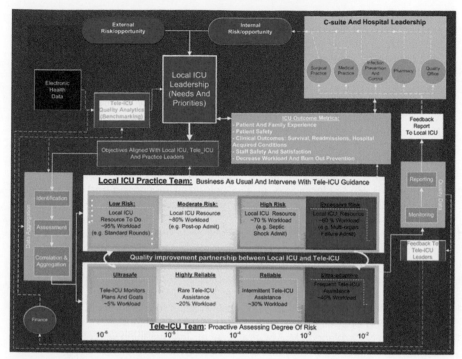

Fig. 3. QI partnership between local ICU and Tele-ICU. C-suite, top senior executives; Tele-ICU, telemedicine intensive care unit.

and after handoff communication might improve clinician preparedness and continuity of care. Tele-ICUs hold standard operating procedures and checklist. As natural language processing technology improves its use during standardized handoff could pre-populate events to be tracked.

SUMMARY

Telemedicine alone does not equate to QI but is merely a tool for QI. The upside is that in the right settings and with the right goals, telemedicine can indeed be used to improve outcomes. Based on the considerations covered here, we recommend that Tele-ICU programs deploy QI methods to monitor process and outcome metrics, and financial impacts closely.

REFERENCES

1. Angus DC, Shorr AF, White A, et al. Critical care delivery in the United States: distribution of services and compliance with Leapfrog recommendations. Crit Care Med 2006;34(4):1016–24.
2. Udeh C, Udeh B, Rahman N, et al. Telemedicine/virtual ICU: where are we and where are we going? Methodist Debakey Cardiovasc J 2018;14(2):126–33.
3. Kahn JM, Cicero BD, Wallace DJ, et al. Adoption of ICU telemedicine in the United States. Crit Care Med 2014;42(2):362–8.
4. Lilly CM, Zubrow MT, Kempner KM, et al. Critical care telemedicine: evolution and state of the art. Crit Care Med 2014;42(11):2429–36.

5. Angus DC, Kelley MA, Schmitz RJ, et al, Committee on Manpower for Pulmonary and Critical Care Societies (COMPACCS). Caring for the critically ill patient. Current and projected workforce requirements for care of the critically ill and patients with pulmonary disease: can we meet the requirements of an aging population? JAMA 2000;284(21):2762-70.

6. Kahn JM. The use and misuse of ICU telemedicine. JAMA 2011;305(21):2227-8.

7. Free from harm. National Patient Safety Foundation.; 2015. p. 59.

8. Vincent C, Amalberti R. Safer healthcare: strategies for the real world. 1st edition. New York: Springer; 2016.

9. Lilly CM, Cody S, Zhao H, et al. Hospital mortality, length of stay, and preventable complications among critically ill patients before and after tele-ICU reengineering of critical care processes. JAMA 2011;305(21):2175-83.

10. Ramnath VR, Ho L, Maggio LA, et al. Centralized monitoring and virtual consultant models of tele-ICU care: a systematic review. Telemed J E Health 2014; 20(10):936-61.

11. Young LB, Chan PS, Lu X, et al. Impact of telemedicine intensive care unit coverage on patient outcomes: a systematic review and meta-analysis. Arch Intern Med 2011;171(6):498-506.

12. Wilcox ME, Adhikari NK. The effect of telemedicine in critically ill patients: systematic review and meta-analysis. Crit Care 2012;16(4):R127.

13. Lilly CM, McLaughlin JM, Zhao H, et al. A multicenter study of ICU telemedicine reengineering of adult critical care. Chest 2014;145(3):500-7.

14. Mackintosh N, Terblanche M, Maharaj R, et al. Telemedicine with clinical decision support for critical care: a systematic review. Syst Rev 2016;5(1):176.

15. Kashani KB, Ramar K, Farmer JC, et al. Quality improvement education incorporated as an integral part of critical care fellows training at the Mayo Clinic. Acad Med 2014;89(10):1362-5.

16. Dilling JA, Swensen SJ, Hoover MR, et al. Accelerating the use of best practices: the Mayo Clinic model of diffusion. Jt Comm J Qual Patient Saf 2013;39(4): 167-76.

17. Iwashyna TJ, Christie JD, Kahn JM, et al. Uncharted paths: hospital networks in critical care. Chest 2009;135(3):827-33.

18. Pannu J, Sanghavi D, Sheley T, et al. Impact of telemedicine monitoring of community ICUs on interhospital transfers. Crit Care Med 2017;45(8):1344-51.

19. Fortis S, Sarrazin MV, Beck BF, et al. ICU telemedicine reduces interhospital ICU transfers in the veterans health administration. Chest 2018;154(1):69-76.

20. Parent B, LaGrone LN, Albirair MT, et al. Effect of standardized handoff curriculum on improved clinician preparedness in the intensive care unit: a stepped-wedge cluster randomized clinical trial. JAMA Surg 2018;153(5):464-70.

Evolution of the Intensive Care Unit Telemedicine Value Proposition

Craig M. Lilly, MD[a,b,*], Jared T. Mickelson, DO[a]

KEYWORDS

- Telemedicine intensive are unit • Case volume • Processes of care • Revenue
- Costs • Direct contribution margin • Financial performance • Outcomes

KEY POINTS

- ICU telemedicine resources are tools for providing evaluation and management services.
- ICU telemedicine programs that improve outcomes change behavior.
- Health care networks can increase their critical care capacity by using ICU telemedicine logistical support.

The value proposition of ICU telemedicine programs is best understood in the context of how the services that they provide are consumed by the organizations that they serve. The deployment of an ICU telemedicine service as passive advice giving support for preexisting services risks adding costs that may be out of proportion to any associated incremental revenue or increased access to critical care services that are provided. Programs that are well integrated into their care-providing ecosystems and provide needed services when and where they are required have been shown to provide financial benefits that substantially exceeded their costs.[1] The financial benefits of providing evaluation and management services and logistical support for the delivery of medical care are generally directly

Conflict of Interest: The author's health care system uses several proprietary electronic systems to provide telemedicine services. None of the authors has received anything of value from any commercial entity relative to the content of this presentation.
[a] Department of Medicine, University of Massachusetts Medical School, Graduate School of Biomedical Sciences, UMass Memorial Health Care, Memorial Medical Center, 55 Lake Avenue North, Worcester, MA 01655, USA; [b] Department of Anesthesiology, and Surgery, Clinical and Population Health Research Program, University of Massachusetts Medical School, Graduate School of Biomedical Sciences, UMass Memorial Health Care, Memorial Medical Center, 281 Lincoln Street, Worcester, MA 01605, USA
* Corresponding author. Departments of Medicine, Anesthesiology, and Surgery, University of Massachusetts Medical School, UMass Memorial Medical Center, 281 Lincoln Street, Worcester, MA 01605.
E-mail address: craig.lilly@umassmed.edu

Crit Care Clin 35 (2019) 463–477
https://doi.org/10.1016/j.ccc.2019.02.010
0749-0704/19/© 2019 Elsevier Inc. All rights reserved.

proportional to the size of the population served. They are directly related to the extent that the ICU telemedicine team uses a leveraged workforce model and can identify and eliminate waste during patient evaluation, management, and transfer processes. ICU telemedicine services have brought value in a growing number of different ways that vary by health care network and by ICU within each network. The primary objective of this presentation is to detail the best-known aspects of ICU telemedicine programs that have brought value as summarized by domain in **Table 1**.

The original implementation of ICU telemedicine services[2] using a passive advice-only model failed in no small part, because steady-state costs exceeded its benefits. Comparison of this failed experiment with its financially successful successor programs has helped to define the elements of telemedicine programs that have been associated with favorable financial performance. The 1970s version of ICU telemedicine consultation involved communication by closed-circuit television that allowed bedside non-specialist physicians to organize and summarize clinical information for review and comment by an off-site intensivist team. The connected hospital clinicians served as the sole source of patient information and could accept, decline, or debate intensivist advice while on camera. The implementation of this telecommunications intensive approach caused great initial satisfaction, as those who provided advice enjoyed the gratitude of the underserved physicians who were excited to learn the fundamentals of delivering critical care services. This initial enthusiasm was followed by a growing realization by the remote hospital physicians that the time required to organize and present cases to the experts could be better spent performing reimbursed care delivery activities. Over time, the intensivists came to feel that the advice they were providing was less appreciated, repeated recently offered recommendations, and could be just as effectively provided by their trainees. Accordingly, they began to be personally present for the telemedicine rounds only on an intermittent basis. The remote hospital physicians perceived that the advice was less frequently useful and varied in its quality; they subsequently only presented cases for whom they had specific questions while the off-site team was unaware of other cases for whom their

Table 1	
Aspects of ICU telemedicine programs that have brought value by domain	
Domain	**Aspects**
Situational Awareness	Early warning systems
	Automated acuity measures
	Transfer readiness tool
Enhanced Communication	Live AV session during episodes of physiologic instability
	Sign in and Sign out
	Escalation pathways
Efficiency Tools	Workforce leveraging
	Economies of scale
	Interprofessional logistical support
	ICU service load balancing
	Reporting Services
Interventions	Real-time encouragement of staff engagement
	Medical management services
	Documentation services
	Incremental staffing support for tasks
	Continuous management of rapidly changing conditions

input would have been helpful. Ultimately the program was closed, because all parties perceived declining and limited value.

It took several decades for the field of ICU telemedicine to develop effective solutions that addressed the inefficient activation characteristics, evolved a more direct and helpful medical management service delivery model, and improved the communication matrix characteristics of the physician-activated advice-only model.

EARLY WARNING SYSTEMS

One key advance was the development of early warning systems that allow off-site providers identify patients with impending physiologic instability using electronic automation that did not require bedside provider action. The ability of standard biomedical monitors alone to accomplish this aim is limited. However, the presence of biomedical monitors that were originally designed to reduce the labor costs of collecting vital sign data and provide continuous displays of electrocardiographic and respiratory parameters enabled the automated prediction of impending physiologic instability. Biomedical monitoring systems that were designed for ICUs displayed signals from several patients on a centrally located ICU monitoring station. Early generation biomedical surveillance systems provided a visual signal from each monitored bed to a dedicated individual who was trained to recognize abnormal cardiac rhythms. This person provided verbal alerts to clinical team members. The effectiveness of these systems depended on the skill of the individual performing the monitoring for correctly identifying actionable abnormalities and on how adroitly they interacted with his or her supporting nurse colleagues who had their competing tasks interrupted. Work interruption-related dissatisfactions and the costs of the individual who provided the monitoring encouraged the development of more extensive and expensive technological solutions.

Biomedical monitor manufacturers added decentralized monitors that also displayed physiologic signals on in-room monitors and added audible alerts to attract the nurse's attention. Dedicated central monitoring workflows gave way to primary monitoring by the patient's nurse. These more expensive systems were attractive, because they lowered the labor costs of monitoring critically ill adults. However, the unintended consequences were that they generated patient complains about noise and created gaps in vigilance when nurses attended to other duties.

Current generation biomedical monitoring systems are deliberately engineered to detect, display, and provide a distinct and easily audible alarm for every episode of physiologic deterioration. The laudable focus on detection of every clinically significant event had the unintended consequence of generating unfortunate numbers of irritating false-positive alerts that interrupt ICU workflows. In addition to bedside audible alarms being a source of patient complaints about noise and sleep disruption, the frequency of false-positive alerts relative to true positive alerts was high enough to cause ICU bedside caregivers to tune-out alerts in a well-recognized and unsafe paradigm known as alarm fatigue.[3,4] The patient safety implications of alarm fatigue were considerable enough for the Joint Commission to focus on alarm management as 2017 national patient safety goal NPSG.06.01.01.[5] Unfortunately, manufacturer-suggested parameter adjustment has not proven to be an effective countermeasure, because it frequently fails to reduce false-positive ICU alarms to patient-friendly and nonprovider annoying levels and often requires amounts of bedside clinician time that are not available.[6]

The broad adoption of these biomedical monitoring systems also facilitated human factor studies of how alerts and alarms impact critical care unit workflows. The results of these studies better define the frequency of safety gaps created by bedside nurse-centered critical care monitoring systems. Interventional studies also demonstrate the value of human curation of system-generated alerts and alarms to reduce false-positive alerts and ensure expeditious recognition and timely responses to episodes of physiologic instability. One key finding reported by these studies is that a typical 15-bed high-acuity adult ICU generated 6.8 true positive (managed with a clinical intervention) alerts each day[7] and that 5 of these alerts were recognized and addressed by the bedside staff.

Unrecognized alarms occurred 1.8 times per day. Each alarm required an off-site critical care professional to prompt the bedside team to address the evolving patient safety risk. Not surprisingly, these nearly missed opportunities for earlier intervention clustered with times that monitoring by critical care nurses was most compromised by competing tasks. It was noted that obtaining medications from dispensing devices, verifying accuracy of blood product administration, attending to the needs of other patients, manipulating life support devices, and participating in end-of-shift or transition of care communication sessions were necessary tasks that competed for the attention of the patient's nurse.

Comprehensive ICU telemedicine programs[8] use early warning systems to cover safety gaps inherent in the bedside nurse-centered patient monitoring model. The 1.8 events per ICU per day frequency of unrecognized impending physiologic instability is a labor increment that is difficult for most ICU-based staffing models to address. Because ICU telemedicine programs provide support to many ICUs, they can provide monitoring solutions at far lower per ICU costs than the former 1 individual performing monitoring for a single ICU model.

INTENSIVE CARE UNIT TELEMEDICINE PATIENT MONITORING SYSTEMS

Understanding the financial implications of eliminating these gaps in vigilance has been facilitated by studies of the epidemiology of adult ICU alerts and alarms.[7,9,10] These studies reported that among critically ill adults, biomedical monitor-based alerts and alarms occurred with equal frequency during daytime and nighttime hours and that weekday and weekend rates were similar. Not surprisingly, rates of episodes of unrecognized physiologic instability that these alarms are designed to detect were lower at times when ICU physician teams were present on the unit. During interprofessional rounding and daytime hours when prescribing providers were scheduled to be on their units, the rates of off-site team-intercepted events were 0.45 events per day. Similar to the findings of studies of nurse biomedical monitor interactions, these events occurred primarily when ICU providers were so focused on current task or procedure completion that they were not cognizant of evolving deterioration among the other ICU patients for whom they were responsible.

Applying mediation analyses to a large verified data set from an ICU telemedicine intervention study,[9] it was estimated that 25% of the length-of-stay benefit of the ICU telemedicine intervention could be accounted for by telemedicine center clinician curation of bedside nurse responses to alerts and alarms. The direct inverse relation of length of stay (LOS) and patient volume allowed the ICU telemedicine intervention to be associated with annual improved financial performance of approximately $700,000 per high-acuity adult ICU.[11]

AUTOMATED ACUITY AND TRANSFER READINESS

Another advance that allows identification of high risk for physiologic instability patients that enables prospective evaluation was the development of systems that identify high-acuity high-mortality risk patients. Automating the identification of these patients allows off-site team members to prospectively review the records of high-risk patients before they develop a physiologic signature of impending deterioration. Conversely, they can identify low-risk patients who may be appropriate for ICU discharge. Electronic systems that prompt discussion of discharge or transfer during interprofessional rounds and before evening sign-out allow off-site providers to be aware of bedside team-identified patients who are appropriate for transfer or discharge. Proper credentialing and access to the electronic record allow the off-site team to provide direct support to bedside providers and reduce delays related to labor-intensive discharge or transfer tasks. The combination of access to the medical record with an early warning system and automated acuity measurement are well-established methods for providing intelligence to off-site team members without interrupting bedside provider workflows. One key element of effective workflows is that they include timely electronic communication among bedside and off-site support team members.

COMMUNICATION FOR TEAM HARMONY AND PATIENT SAFETY

The common thread of successful telemedicine support is timely and effective communication matrices. Successful ICU telemedicine programs are part of the caregiving ecosystem of the ICUs that they serve, and ICU telemedicine providers must communicate effectively with their bedside partners. Although bedside providers appreciate the convenience of not having to ask for help, they strongly disapprove of not being engaged in important management decisions. For this reason, ICU telemedicine programs use a flexible palate of communications methods including secure text messaging, e-mail, electronic notes in the medical record, nonarchival messages embedded in the electronic health record, video conferencing, communication with available team members, and telephone calls. ICU telemedicine staff tailoring of communication with awareness of bedside provider communication preferences is fundamental to effective, timely, and efficient communication. Tuned communication methods allow bedside provider workflow to be interrupted for emergent critical decisions while allowing their off-site coverage to manage noncritical and nonemergent events with their review at a time when their workflow or sleep will not be interrupted. Efficient communication that respects the bedside provider as the director of important decisions and supports their preferred method of communication is key for building the team harmony that allows shared performance goals to be achieved. Organized and regular service sign-out is 1 method that builds relationships, trust, and helps providers get communication right.

INTENSIVE CARE UNIT TELEMEDICINE SIGN-IN AND -OUT PROCEDURES ENHANCE SITUATIONAL AWARENESS

An increasingly common feature of ICU telemedicine services is that they take sign-out from bedside ICU providers at times when they are not present on the ICU.[10] Electronic support[12] for standardized sign-in and sign-out procedures[13–15] is increasingly recognized as more effective than unstructured verbal-only or no sign-out.[16] Not surprisingly, studies of recall after verbal attending sign-out have revealed unfortunate numbers of inaccuracies when human memory alone is relied upon.[17] Access to the electronic medical record has dramatically improved the efficiency of sign-in and sign-out episodes and provides an electronic scaffold upon which accurate information can be efficiently shared and reviewed. Recorded observations of ICU telemedicine sign-in and -out sessions with coding of their content allowed identification of a modest number of common transactional themes.[7] Identification of these themes led to the development of drop-down lists of uncompleted tasks and a way to share less well-developed clinical concerns about risks for near-term instability as part of a standardized sign-out template. Bedside provider sign-out to the ICU telemedicine team also provides an opportunity to identify improving patients who are ready or may soon be ready for transfer, and to communicate off-hours management goals. Electronic sign-out followed by verbal communication is an effective way to document that accurate information was passed among team members. It also enables engagement of the ICU telemedicine team, because it identifies the time at which the first call for clinical issues or attending physician-level questions should go to off-site team members.

DELIVERING MEDICAL MANAGEMENT AND DOCUMENTATION SERVICES: MORE THAN ADVICE

The keystone difference between older advice-only and current generation service providers is the ability to deliver bedside provider support in the form of patient evaluation services and support for required patient care tasks. These services include the recording of provider orders for medications, manipulation of life support devices, arranging and interpreting imaging and laboratory testing, requesting specialist consultation, and arranging necessary procedures. Because off-site team members cannot perform airway stabilization and vascular access procedures, these services are provided by hospital-based procedure teams or by bedside team providers before they sign-out.

Episodes of unplanned life-threatening physiologic deterioration frequently require more interventions than a single bedside nurse can perform unassisted. Off-site critical care professionals provide support during a crisis by prescribing and performing communication services that shorten the time to critical medication or blood product administration, arrange the delivery of life support devices, or hasten the arrival of additional personnel. Empowering the off-site intensivist to communicate with interventional proceduralists or surgical service providers allows bedside personnel to focus on applying advanced life support, performing emergent resuscitation, and evaluating the effectiveness of on-going resuscitation efforts. In addition, their training and access to the electronic health record allow off-site critical care professionals to provide support with timely and correct event documentation.

PATHWAYS FOR ESCALATION

A common theme of retrospective adverse event analyses[18] is that both the request for and arrival of additional resources could have been more timely. Trained and credentialed critical care specialists are directed to acutely deteriorating and highest acuity cases by ICU telemedicine system early warning and automated acuity measuring systems. Continuous real-time availability allows additional evaluation for at-risk patients in whom highe- order cognitive processes are required to reexamine assumptions and for whom specialist experience may allow phenotypic recognition of diseases that have not presented with typical manifestations. Importantly, because off-site team members are less task-focused and work in a less emotionally charged and pressured environment, they less frequently hesitate when additional resources should be mobilized or when the involvement of senior clinicians can provide needed support.

WORKFORCE LEVERAGING

The ability to provide dedicated monitoring over many ICUs makes ICU telemedicine systems a financially attractive option for providing just-in-time additional resources.

In this model, the costs of critical care professionals to prevent missed interventions, improve communication matrices, and deliver emergently needed interventions are spread over a larger number of patients. Technologies that target these services by physiologic indicators provide a safety net at lower per-patient costs than approaches that use time-based or indiscriminate methods of delivery. One indication that off-site support teams are better equipped than off-unit on-call providers is that ICU telemedicine providers are at workstations at times when on-call service providers are engaged in off-screen activities.

ICU telemedicine centers that employ a workforce-leveraged interprofessional team approach provide services where all interprofessional team members practice to the limits of their licensed and credentialed roles. The payer costs for adult critically ill patients managed with Tele-ICU center supervised Advanced Practice Providers (APPs) was significantly less than the costs of concurrent cases managed with traditional ICU staffing models.[19] Management over a regional or larger scale allows one telemedicine intensivist to concurrently supervise the activities of intensivist extenders including hospitalists and APPs at many hospitals, achieving far greater efficiency than on-site only intensivist staffing models can attain.[20,21] One true value of ICU telemedicine programs is that they provide health care networks with flexible and practical access to leveraged critical care workforce models.

A hub and spoke ICU telemedicine program is a currently available way for a health care network to provide high-quality adult critical care services across a broader encashment area.[21] High-acuity patients who have airway stabilization and intravascular access procedures at regional hospital emergency departments can receive high-quality critical care services from hospitalists and APPs[19,22] at the hospital where they presented when the support of a telemedicine intensive care specialist is available. ICU telemedicine support, particularly off-hours support, has allowed smaller hospitals to recruit and retain the on-hours intensivists who allow them to keep their ICUs open. External financial auditing has confirmed that the case revenue from retaining these higher-acuity cases substantially exceeded the costs of the ICU telemedicine support.[22]

INCREMENTAL STAFFING RESOURCES FOR NASCENT PHYSIOLOGIC INSTABILITY

Akin to the individuals who watched the screens of the original on-ICU biomedical monitoring systems, off-site critical care professionals identify true positive alerts and ensure that bedside providers have responded. ICU telemedicine system predictive modeling allows prospective identification of signatures of impending physiologic deterioration. Pre-event notification of dedicated off-site team members allows interrogation of the clinical record and identification of preventable causes in a prospective urgent rather than a retrospective reactive paradigm, encourages team discussion before the time of crisis, ensures that instability is responded to in a timely manner, and provides an additional real-time pathway for escalation. Studies to date suggest that identifying and acting on these opportunities are associated with reduced duration of critical illness[23] and lower numbers of adult critical care medicolegal claims.[20]

TEAMWORK FOR CONTINUOUS MANAGEMENT

ICU telemedicine support is a practical way to transform an interprofessional episodic rounding model to a continuous model of care plan modification that can recognize and immediately support patients with rapidly changing care needs. In this model, bedside intensivists identify therapeutic goals or specific tasks, or follow-up on delegated tasks for their off-site colleagues to perform at times when they are attending to other tasks or are not on the unit. This level of teamwork requires sign-out, established trusting relationships, efficient and effective communication, and true sharing of control and responsibility for outcomes. The ability to identify patients who can benefit from active off-hours management and coordinate the required interprofessional collaboration to accomplish it have been associated with significantly shorter duration of critical illness or injury.[9] Indeed, workstation-assisted intensivist review of off-hours cases within 1 hour of ICU admission was 1 aspect of ICU telemedicine implementation that identified programs with larger reductions in ICU LOS.[23] The common theme of the aspects of ICU telemedicine implementations that were directly associated with shorter LOS in a multicenter study was the ability of ICU teams to work together on well-defined goals using accurate and timely ICU telemedicine program-generated reports.[23]

The benefits of an ICU telemedicine program depends on how efficiently the additional resources are used. A study at a large health care system compared alternative methods of leveraging ICU telemedicine services. ICUs that required ICU telemedicine team members to request that a bedside team member record provider orders were compared with ICUs that had ICU telemedicine team members take immediate action and inform bedside providers of the event in a timely manner. The method of direct action by ICU telemedicine team members was reported to be more efficient, because it was associated with shorter LOS.[24]

AN INTERPROFESSIONAL APPROACH TO LOGISTICAL SUPPORT

Variation of the services that are available among the medical centers serving a region has led to a paradigm in which patient transfers are increasingly common. Virtually every site at which medical care is provided will make or receive requests for the interfacility transfer of patients. The issue is not whether medical centers provide logistical services; rather it is how efficiently they provide them. The traditional approach of having hospital operators direct calls to on-call physicians has given way at most medical centers to dedicated referral phone numbers to that are triaged by individuals with clinical training. The advent of telemedicine centers with multiscreen workstations and interprofessional staff trained in the care of high-acuity patients has led to a leveraged workforce approach to reducing wait times for clinicians requesting referrals and shorter arrival times for patients. The ICU telemedicine center can expedite physician case acceptance while encouraging resuscitation, expediting time-sensitive diagnostics, and reducing postreferral center arrival delays.

DECREASED TIME TO RESCUE

Logistical support has 2 main functions. The first is to reduce the time to urgently required interventions, and the second is to increase access to high-quality care. Making telemedicine center expertise and best practice protocols available to those managing patients requiring time-sensitive therapies is increasingly seen as more efficient than management without support. ICU telemedicine center access to the electronic health and radiographic records and the ability to view and interview patients on camera have revolutionized stroke care.[25] Recent advances allow this experience also to be available to other critically ill patients waiting in emergency departments (EDs). A recent study reported that patients receiving ICU telemedicine support in the ED during times when patient volume has exceeded ED provider capacity had lower mortality and less frequently required ICU admission than patients not receiving ICU telemedicine center-supported care.[26] Another example of the role of ICU telemedicine for time-sensitive care is ICU telemedicine center support for patients presenting with sepsis. Patients presenting to an ED with sepsis were identified and received potentially lifesaving therapies[27] sooner when ICU telemedicine nurses provided standardized screening and facilitated interventions than when sepsis detection was done primarily by ED clinical staff.[28]

LOGISTICAL SUPPORT TO INCREASED ACCESS TO CARE

ICU telemedicine program logistical support has also increased access to critical care services.[11,22] Access to critical care services is expanded by decreasing ICU LOS, identifying and tapping unused ICU capacity, and creating ICU capacity by enhancing patient flow. Well-implemented ICU telemedicine programs reduce the LOS,[23] in part by improving adherence to ICU best practice guidelines.[9,29] Financial analyses of an ICU telemedicine program implementation have identified a near mirror image (indirect) relationship of LOS and annual ICU patient volume,[11] while reports of implementations without impact on LOS have not found financial benefits.[30] ICU telemedicine program logistical support also increased patient volume by displaying unused ICU capacity to an off-site intensivist who was empowered to facilitate the transfer of appropriate patients to those available beds. Telemedicine program support can also create capacity by facilitating the off-hours transfer or discharge of patients who have been identified by their bedside attending physician as ready for discharge. In addition, telemedicine systems with predictive analytical support can create bed capacity by identifying tasks like physical or occupational therapy evaluations, radiographic studies, insurance reviews, and family concerns that can be attended to before the anticipated day of discharge.

FINANCIAL PERFORMANCE: A MATTER OF PERSPECTIVE

The interpretation of financial performance metrics depends on funds flow perspective. Costs of providing access borne by patients, families, and payers are viewed as revenue for providers and hospitals, **Fig. 1**.

From the point of view of patients and families, ICU telemedicine logistical support reduces wait times and allows more patients to be cared for at a hospital that is close to the patient's home. Financial benefits of closer-to-home care include lower lodging, parking, and transportation costs that families must bear. In addition, video access to their intensivist and specialists is a valued and increasingly expected service that connects patients and their families to the institutions that care for them.

From the point of view of the prescribing provider, ICU telemedicine is a resource that can increase individual productivity, because off-site providers can provide support for documentation and other tasks that can divert bedside providers toward more fulfilling and productive activities. Logistical support is particularly valued, because bedside providers rely on off-site colleagues to manage bed request calls, assist with transfer electronic paperwork, and provide low-risk prescribing and out-of-rounds clinical evaluations for bedside providers. Changing the environment to better support uninterrupted focus on individual critically ill patients is 1 way to improve the patient and provider experience.[31]

Early warning systems allow qualified and credentialed colleagues to help bedside providers identify care opportunities that require immediate bedside presence and to perform tasks for them at times when it is better not to interrupt them. Not surprisingly, surveys of ICU nurses have documented a preference for immediate telemedicine access to intensivist expertise[32] and for the help and advice of more experienced nursing colleagues.[33–35] The ability of telemedicine programs to add qualified and credentialed person power at times when local clinical workload has exceeded workforce

Patient Perspective
- Right care
- Right place
-Right time
- Shorter wait times
- Lower family lodging
and parking costs
with referal medical center
expertise closer to home

Provider Perspective
- Help with logistical tasks
- Help getting the MD to the bedside
- Help with prescribing tasks
-Person power when urgent tasks
exceed provider capacity
-Lower burnout rates
- More time for financial productivity

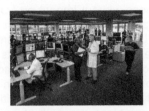

ICU Telemedicine Program
Interprofessional Logistical Support

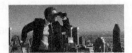

Healthcare Network Perspective
-Shorter length of stay
- Increased volume
- Tapping unused capacity

Payer Perspective
- Lower costs for lower acuity patients
- Lower transportaion costs
- Improved access to specialized care

Fig. 1. Financial benefits of operational efficiency changes related to ICU telemedicine program logistical support from the patient, ICU provider, health care system, and payer perspectives.

capacity is a potent countermeasure for the phenomenon of burnout that threatens the critical care workforce.[36,37]

From the point of view of hospitals that provide advanced specialized services and procedures, the financial benefits of ICU telemedicine relate to reducing the LOS and increasing the volume of cases that benefit from the advanced specialized care that they are designed to provide. ICU telemedicine programs reduce LOS by providing critical care professionals that recognize and respond to episodes of physiologic instability earlier and achieve near-perfect adherence to consensus ICU best practices.[29] The logistical support that they provide increases and optimizes the use of their ICU capacity and benefits patients by more quickly providing access the critical care services that they require at locations that are more frequently near their homes.[9,11,23] Early recognition, intervention, and logistical services have been associated with sustained annual increases of case volume of 38%, with relatively flat costs per case, and with a 450% improvement of direct contribution margin. The costs of

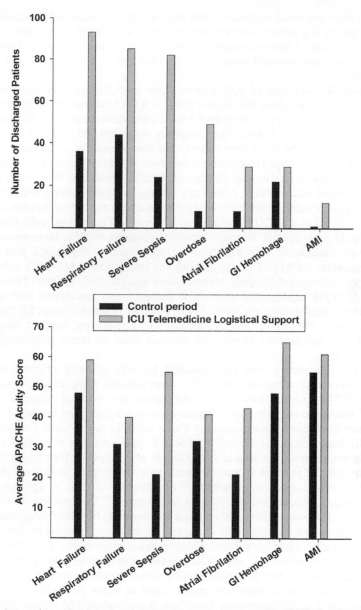

Fig. 2. Patient volume (top) and average acuity score (bottom) by MS-DRG group. MS DRGs 922, 918, 871, 378, 377, 317, 310, 309, 293, 292, 291, 280, 281,208, 207, 189, and 177 were grouped by ICU diagnosis after consolidation across payers. (*Adapted from* Fifer S, Everett W, Adams M, et al, Massachusetts Technology Collaborative, New England Healthcare Institute. Critical care, critical choices the case for tele-ICUs in intensive care. Cambridge (MA): New England Healthcare Institute; Massachusetts Technology Collaborative; 2010. p. 54. Available at: https://www.nehi.net/publications/19-critical-care-critical-choices-the-case-for-tele-icus-in-intensive-care/view.)

implementation are small compared with the benefits of improved financial performance when the implementation is associated with a more efficient critical care service delivery model.[11] One key enabler of enhanced medical center performance is accurate, timely, and relevant reports with metrics tied to benchmarks and relevant comparators.

The financial outcomes of ICU telemedicine and logistical services program implementation for hospitals that do not provide a full spectrum of medical services have been reported by an independent health care institute after verification by an external auditing firm.[22] Subscribing hospitals were able to care for significantly more critically ill adults when their teams had the support of an off-site qualified, credentialed, and privileged to practice intensivist. Stratification by discharge Medicare Severity Diagnosis Related Groups (MS-DRG) indicated that more patients with sepsis, heart failure shock, pulmonary edema, cardiac arrhythmias, drug overdose, and gastrointestinal (GI) hemorrhage were cared for at the hospital that they presented to during the ICU telemedicine intervention compared with the control period (Fig. 2). In addition to increasing patient volumes, the ICU telemedicine intervention was associated with significantly higher acute physiology and chronic health evaluation (APACHE) acuity scores for nearly every MS-DRG category.[22] Accordingly, subscribed hospital revenue was substantially greater, because the retention of higher-acuity adult critically ill patients was associated with a significantly higher hospital case mix index (CMI). Another notable change for these hospitals was that the immediate availability of high-quality support when their intensivist was not present in the ICU allowed them to retain their local critical care specialists.

The payer perspective also has revealed benefits of more efficient care and logistical processes observed after ICU telemedicine program implementation. Studies,[33,38–40] including those with verification by external financial auditing firms,[19,22] have reported that more efficient care paradigms bring benefits to payers. Federal and nonfederal payers seeking these benefits have made investments to create ICU telemedicine services.[30,41] Cost of care analyses were performed by comparing the payer's expenses of 449 patients who stayed at their presenting hospital to the costs of patients sent to a referral medical center. Costs were measured using activity-based accounting methods[42] for patients matched by age, gender, primary discharge ICD code, and APACHE III acuity score.[22] The average inpatient hospitalization costs borne by third-party payers of presenting hospital management were $10,000 per case less than the costs of cases sent to referral medical centers. In addition, payers and families bore incremental transportation costs. Calculation of the financial benefits of effectively using ICU telemedicine tools to manage ICU logistics across Massachusetts identified meaningful financial improvements for payers. Using the average difference of usual care payer costs to those of the ICU telemedicine group from the 2 study community hospitals, a state-wide 122 million (2011 USD) lower financial burden was calculated.[22] Current regional referral and local support models for critically ill and injured adults are not logistically optimized.

SUMMARY

Advances in clinical information sciences, telecommunication technologies, electronic health records, early warning systems, automated acuity assessment, and clinician communication support systems have allowed current-generation ICU telemedicine systems to address the inefficiencies of the failed advice-upon-request ICU telemedicine model. Value is related to the ability of health care systems to leverage ICU telemedicine resources to provide care when and where their high-acuity patients need evaluation and management services. Local financial benefits of ICU telemedicine program implementation depend on changing behavior to better focus on activities that reduce the duration of critical illness and LOS. Financial outcomes for health care networks and payers are also related to more efficient logistical management that identifies and taps unused critical care capacity and creates additional capacity using existing resources.

ACKNOWLEDGMENTS

The authors express their gratitude for the ongoing and tireless support of the UMass Memorial Healthcare Critical Care Operations members.

REFERENCES

1. Lilly CM, Motzkus CA. ICU telemedicine: financial analyses of a complex intervention. Crit Care Med 2017;45(9):1558–61.
2. Grundy BL, Crawford P, Jones PK, et al. Telemedicine in critical care: an experiment in health care delivery. JACEP 1977;6(10):439–44.
3. Johnson KR, Hagadorn JI, Sink DW. Alarm safety and alarm fatigue. Clin Perinatol 2017;44(3):713–28.
4. Winters BD, Cvach MM, Bonafide CP, et al. Technological distractions (part 2): a summary of approaches to manage clinical alarms with intent to reduce alarm fatigue. Crit Care Med 2018;46(1):130–7.
5. Commission J. National patient safety goals effective January 2017 - Joint Commission. Joint Commission; 2017.
6. Kane-Gill SL, O'Connor MF, Rothschild JM, et al. Technologic distractions (part 1): summary of approaches to manage alert quantity with intent to reduce alert fatigue and suggestions for alert fatigue metrics. Crit Care Med 2017;45(9): 1481–8.
7. Lilly CM, Thomas EJ. Tele-ICU: experience to date. J Intensive Care Med 2010; 25(1):16–22.
8. Reynolds HN, Sheinfeld G, Chang J, et al. The tele-intensive care unit during a disaster: seamless transition from routine operations to disaster mode. Telemed J E Health 2011;17(9):746–9.
9. Lilly CM, Cody S, Zhao H, et al. Hospital mortality, length of stay, and preventable complications among critically ill patients before and after tele-ICU reengineering of critical care processes. JAMA 2011;305(21):2175–83.
10. Lilly CM, Fisher KA, Ries M, et al. A national ICU telemedicine survey: validation and results. Chest 2012;142(1):40–7.
11. Lilly CM, Motzkus C, Rincon T, et al. ICU telemedicine program financial outcomes. Chest 2017;151(2):286–97.
12. Nemeth C, Nunnally M, O'Connor M, et al. Creating resilient IT: how the sign-out sheet shows clinicians make healthcare work. AMIA Annu Symp Proc 2006;584–8.
13. Nanchal R, Aebly B, Graves G, et al. Controlled trial to improve resident sign-out in a medical intensive care unit. BMJ Qual Saf 2017;26(12):987–92.
14. Lee JC, Horst M, Rogers A, et al. Checklist-styled daily sign-out rounds improve hospital throughput in a major trauma center. Am Surg 2014;80(5):434–40.
15. Emlet LL, Al-Khafaji A, Kim YH, et al. Trial of shift scheduling with standardized sign-out to improve continuity of care in intensive care units. Crit Care Med 2012;40(12):3129–34.

16. Raduma-Tomas MA, Flin R, Yule S, et al. Doctors' handovers in hospitals: a literature review. BMJ Qual Saf 2011;20(2):128–33.

17. Dutra M, Monteiro M, Ribeiro K, et al. Handovers among staff intensivists. Crit Care Med 2018;46(11):1717–21.

18. Anderson CI, Nelson CS, Graham CF, et al. Disorganized care: the findings of an iterative, in-depth analysis of surgical morbidity and mortality. J Surg Res 2012; 177(1):43–8.

19. Trombley MJ, Hassol A, Lloyd JT, et al. The impact of enhanced critical care training and 24/7 (tele-ICU) support on Medicare spending and postdischarge utilization patterns. Health Serv Res 2018;53(4):20992117.

20. Lilly CM, Zubrow MT, Kempner KM, et al. Critical care telemedicine: evolution and state of the art. Crit Care Med 2014;42(11):2429–36.

21. Groves RH Jr, Holcomb BW Jr, Smith ML. Intensive care telemedicine: evaluating a model for proactive remote monitoring and intervention in the critical care setting. Stud Health Technol Inform 2008;131:131–46.

22. Fifer S, Everett W, Adams M, et al, Massachusetts Technology Collaborative, New England Healthcare Institute. Critical care, critical choices the case for tele-ICUs in intensive care. Cambridge (MA): New England Healthcare Institute; Massachusetts Technology Collaborative; 2010. Available at: http://www.masstech.org/teleICU.pdf.

23. Lilly CM, McLaughlin JM, Zhao H, et al. A multicenter study of ICU telemedicine reengineering of adult critical care. Chest 2014;145(3):500–7.

24. Hawkins HA, Lilly CM, Kaster DA, et al. ICU telemedicine comanagement methods and length of stay. Chest 2016;150(2):314–9.

25. Dorsey ER, Glidden AM, Holloway MR, et al. Teleneurology and mobile technologies: the future of neurological care. Nat Rev Neurol 2018;14(5):285–97.

26. Kadar RB, AD, Hesse K, et al. Impact of telemonitoring of critically ill emergency department patients awaiting intensive care unit transfer. Crit Care Med, in press.

27. Rhodes A, Evans LE, Alhazzani W, et al. Surviving sepsis campaign: international guidelines for management of sepsis and septic shock: 2016. Crit Care Med 2017;45(3):486–552.

28. Rincon TA, Manos EL, Pierce JD. Telehealth intensive care unit nurse surveillance of sepsis. Comput Inform Nurs 2017;35(9):459–64.

29. Kahn JM, Gunn SR, Lorenz HL, et al. Impact of nurse-led remote screening and prompting for evidence-based practices in the ICU*. Crit Care Med 2014;42(4): 896–904.

30. Nassar BS, Vaughan-Sarrazin MS, Jiang L, et al. Impact of an intensive care unit telemedicine program on patient outcomes in an integrated health care system. JAMA Intern Med 2014;174(7):1160–7.

31. Moss M, Good VS, Gozal D, et al. An official critical care societies collaborative statement-burnout syndrome in critical care health-care professionals: a call for action. Chest 2016;150(1):17–26.

32. Chu-Weininger MY, Wueste L, Lucke JF, et al. The impact of a tele-ICU on provider attitudes about teamwork and safety climate. Qual Saf Health Care 2010; 19(6):e39.

33. Goran SF. A second set of eyes: an introduction to tele-ICU. Crit Care Nurse 2010; 30(4):46–55 [quiz: 56].

34. Romig MC, Latif A, Gill RS, et al. Perceived benefit of a telemedicine consultative service in a highly staffed intensive care unit. J Crit Care 2012;27(4):426.e9-16.

35. Ward MM, Ullrich F, Potter AJ, et al. Factors affecting staff perceptions of tele-ICU service in rural hospitals. Telemed J E Health 2015;21(6):459–66.

36. Angus DC, Kelley MA, Schmitz RJ, et al. Caring for the critically ill patient. Current and projected workforce requirements for care of the critically ill and patients with pulmonary disease: can we meet the requirements of an aging population? JAMA 2000;284(21):2762–70.
37. Moss M, Good VS, Gozal D, et al. An official critical care societies collaborative statement: burnout syndrome in critical care healthcare professionals: a call for action. Crit Care Med 2016;44(7):1414–21.
38. Zawada ET Jr, Herr P, Larson D, et al. Impact of an intensive care unit telemedicine program on a rural health care system. Postgrad Med 2009;121(3):160–70.
39. Goran SF. Making the move: from bedside to camera-side. Crit Care Nurse 2012; 32(1):e20–9.
40. Cowboy E, Simmons R, Miller S, et al. Preventing air embolisms with tele-ICU collaborative. Chest Journal 2009;136(4):16S.
41. Blue Cross of California gets $1.8 million for rural telemedicine program. Telemed Virtual Real 1998;3(12):135.
42. Udpa S. Activity cost analysis: a tool to cost medical services and improve quality of care. Manag Care Q 2001;9(3):34–41.

Intensive Care Unit Telemedicine Care Models

Sean M. Caples, DO, MS

KEYWORDS

- Tele-ICU • Telemedicine • Intensive care • e-ICU • Care models

KEY POINTS

- Tele-ICU care can be delivered with as few as 1 intensivist. Nurses and advanced practice providers, as well as administrative support are commonly part of the care team.
- Care models can be classified as high or low intensity, as they relate to the domains of time, scope, interaction with the bedside staff, and whether care is more proactive or reactive.
- Tele-ICU can be often be successfully used as an educational model for trainees.

INTRODUCTION

Since its first description in 1977,[1] when interactive television was used by intensivists to provide consultation to physicians staffing a community hospital, telemedicine monitoring of intensive care units (tele-ICU) is increasingly used as a model to care for patients who are critically ill. Bolstered by more sophisticated technology, care models have evolved over the past 4 decades as the use of tele-ICU has expanded, with estimates that in excess of 15% of ICU beds in the United States are covered by such programs.[2] Models of ICU telemedicine care can vary in a number of ways, from the composition and coverage hours of the monitoring hub to the level of involvement with the patients and local staff.[3,4]

BASIC PRINCIPLES

Tele-ICU models can be simply conceptualized by distinguishing the tele-ICU specialists who monitor and deliver care from the remotely located patients and care team receiving the support elsewhere. This can be traditionally defined by the "hub and spoke" model, in which the tele-ICU specialists operate out of a centralized location, which typically also houses computers, specialized software, and monitoring equipment.[5] Alternatively, because the technology offers flexibility, the tele-ICU specialists

No financial disclosures.

The Enhanced Critical Care Program, Division of Pulmonary and Critical Care Medicine, Mayo Clinic, 200 First Street Southwest, Rochester, MN 55905, USA

E-mail address: caples.sean@mayo.edu

can be dispersed virtually anywhere that has a reliable and secure Internet connection, including offices or even homes.

When considering human resourcing, in its simplest form, tele-ICU care may be delivered by a single specialist, usually an intensivist. More commonly, and sometimes in order to scale to a level that can promote financial solvency (if not profit), staffing often includes critical care trained nurses and sometimes advanced practice providers (such as nurse practitioners or physician assistants). Ancillary personnel can provide administrative support for higher resourced programs. Industry-standard ratios approximate 1 physician to approximately 100 patients and 1 nurse for every 30 or 40 patients, assuming that the tasks of populating tele-ICU software as well as the bulk of charting responsibilities fall to the tele-ICU nurse.

INTENSITY OF THE CARE MODELS

Beyond the members of the care team, tele-ICU systems might be stratified by the intensity in which care is provided. A high-intensity tele-ICU care model might be defined by 24-hours-a-day monitoring of every bed in an ICU, whereas a lower-intensity model of care might be limited to a portion of a 24-hour period, most commonly the overnight hours, or monitoring of a selected proportion of beds in an ICU. Such decisions on workflows and practice modeling are typically made jointly between the telemedicine team and hospital being monitored, depending on the needs for patient care (**Table 1**).

High-intensity monitoring might also be defined by a proactive approach to patient care. This model might include assessments of new admissions within a specified period of time (for example, within 30 or 60 minutes), in-depth chart review, and assurance of application of evidence-based, best-practice critical care medicine, including adherence to all elements of care bundles. The tele-ICU team might take an active and longitudinal role in the care of the remote patient, with ordering laboratory and imaging tests and prescribing medications or changes in mechanical ventilation settings. Daily progress notes might be written in the chart, akin to a formal consulting service. The tele-intensivist can conduct video rounds in the patient room, and in some instances might incorporate the bedside nurse and/or a member of the local care provider team, including the primary physician. It is not uncommon to engage family members who may have questions about care or prognosis. In a proactive model, nursing assessments, including video interaction, are often scheduled routinely (for example, every

Table 1 Elements of higher-intensity and lower-intensity tele–intensive care unit (tele-ICU) care models	
Higher-Intensity Tele-ICU	**Lower-Intensity Tele-ICU**
Continuous (24-h) coverage	Discontinuous (12–16-h) coverage
Multiple layers of critical care personnel (intensivist, critical care nurse, advance practice providers, ancillary personnel for administrative duties)	As few as 1 person (intensivist)
Proactive approach (round on every patient, chart review, alter/prescribe treatments and plan of care to promote best practice)	Reactive approach (respond to automated acuity alerts or emergencies)
Daily progress notes, longitudinal care of all patients	Documentation with interventions as needed on specific patients
Quality reports, benchmarking	

12 hours). Although such activities are not necessarily exclusive of a discontinuous (nighttime-only) model of care, 24 hours a day continuous monitoring promotes a proactive approach to patient care.

A low-intensity monitoring tele-ICU might be characterized by a reactive (or less proactive) model of care. Tele-ICU involvement might be limited to responding to software alarms indicating abnormal vital signs or aberrant physiologic parameters as they occur. Video assessments or treatment interventions might be limited to instances when assistance or consultation is requested by the local care providers or nurses. Some hospitals are staffed by an intensivist who is present during the day but not at night; a low-intensity model might be appropriate.

When creating workflows, it is essential to highlight the fact that the onset of an acute event such as an arrhythmia or cardiopulmonary arrest will not be immediately apparent to the tele-ICU team, because there is a delay in data acquisition and analysis before funneling to the software interface that is viewed by the tele-ICU staff. Therefore, direct communication between the bedside team and the tele-ICU operations center is essential in an emergency. Although this can be accomplished by telephone, it can be more efficiently used by a digital alert system connecting the patient room to the software in the tele-ICU hub.

Many tele-ICU programs are designed within the framework of a regional health system governed by a single institution.[6] An example would be a tele-ICU hub based at the tertiary care center and the spokes represented by community-based ICUs that generally "feed" to the tertiary center for specialty care of more complex cases. Direct communication between the tele-ICU, emergency departments, and often a centralized telecommunications center allows more precise and intentional control of ICU bed occupancy across a regional system, and also promotes dissemination of a standardized approach to the critically ill patient across that system. Such a practice allows movement of sicker patients to more resourced ICUs within the system.[7] However, the usual tenet that tele-ICU programs allow for better retention of ICU patients remaining at their community hospital might not apply to this model. A recent study of a regional health system showed that, following implementation of a tele-ICU program, interhospital transfers from the community to the tertiary center actually increased compared with the rate of transfers before the program launch,[8] a finding that was not explained by an increase in overall severity of illness. It is hypothesized that, within an integrated health system, a *transfer bias* partially drives such findings.

QUALITY IMPROVEMENT

Tele-ICU programs that provide comprehensive service, through data acquisition and analysis, often provide quality metrics on a periodic basis. Such data can serve to benchmark against other programs and peer institutions and provide a foundation for quality improvement projects.

The tele-ICU is also a rich environment to foster nursing quality initiatives. The usually experienced critical care nurses who staff ICU telemedicine programs can offer valuable mentorship to less experienced bedside nurses.

INTENSIVE CARE UNIT TELEMEDICINE AS A MODEL FOR MEDICAL EDUCATION

There may be a theoretic concern that the autonomy and, therefore, the experiential education of medical trainees might be eroded by the presence of an ICU telemedicine program.[9,10] In theory, a resident or fellow might behave deferentially or defensively in medical decision-making with the knowledge that a consulting intensivist is involved in the case at hand, even with a concern for micromanagement on the part of the telemedicine providers. On the other hand, there is an argument that early warning system software used in ICU telemedicine would serve as a useful platform for the tele-intensivist to educate learners on the assessment of the deteriorating patient. Similarly, it might be considered an added advantage that the tele-intensivist is available to the trainee during off hours. In addition to reviewing clinical data and management plans, tele-intensivists also can provide guidance and instruction on bedside procedures.

Limited published data based on surveys of medical learners generally report favorable views of ICU telemedicine programs, citing improvements in patient care and safety and a willingness or even desire to learn within the framework of such tele-ICU programs.[11]

SUMMARY

Various care models can satisfy the needs of many ICU practices in search of tele-ICU partnership.[12] Determinants include infrastructure, local governance, and acuity. The cost of a high-intensity model may be justified for some practices; others may be well served by lower-intensity tele-ICU care.

REFERENCES

1. Grundy BL, Jones PK, Lovitt A. Telemedicine in critical care: problems in design, implementation, and assessment. Crit Care Med 1982;10:471–5.
2. Kahn JM, Cicero BD, Wallace DJ, et al. Adoption of ICU telemedicine in the United States. Crit Care Med 2014;42:362–8.
3. Lilly CM, Fisher KA, Ries M, et al. A national ICU telemedicine survey: validation and results. Chest 2012;142:40–7.
4. L. H. S. R. Series. ICU physician staffing. Available at: URL|. Accessed Access Date, Access Year|.
5. Vranas.KC, Slatore CG, Kerlin MP. Telemedicine coverage of intensive care units: a narrative review. Ann Am Thorac Soc 2018. https://doi.org/10.1513/AnnalsATS.201804-225FR.
6. Nassar BS, Vaughan-Sarrazin MS, Jiang L, et al. Impact of an intensive care unit telemedicine program on patient outcomes in an integrated health care system. JAMA Intern Med 2014;174:1160–7.
7. Fortis S, Sarrazin MV, Beck BF, et al. ICU telemedicine reduces interhospital ICU transfers in the Veterans Health Administration. Chest 2018;154:69–76.
8. Pannu J, Sanghavi D, Sheley T, et al. Impact of telemedicine monitoring of community ICUs on interhospital transfers. Crit Care Med 2017;45:1344–51.
9. Coletti C, Elliott DJ, Zubrow MT. Resident perceptions of a tele-intensive care unit implementation. Telemed J E Health 2010;16:894–7.
10. Summe A, Foor L, Hoeck L, et al. Resident perceptions of competency and comfort before and after telemedicine-ICU implementation. South Med J 2018;111:344–7.
11. Lilly CM, Zubrow MT, Kempner KM, et al. Critical care telemedicine: evolution and state of the art. Crit Care Med 2014;42:2429–36.
12. Hawkins HA, Lilly CM, Kaster DA, et al. ICU telemedicine comanagement methods and length of stay. Chest 2016;150:314–9.

Intensive Care Unit Telemedicine in the Era of Big Data, Artificial Intelligence, and Computer Clinical Decision Support Systems

Ryan D. Kindle, MD[a,b,1], Omar Badawi, PharmD, MPH, FCCM[a,c,d,2],
Leo Anthony Celi, MD, MS, MPH[a,b,*,1],
Shawn Sturland, MBChB, FANZCA, FCICM[a,e,1]

KEYWORDS

- Telemedicine • ICU • Machine learning • Clinical decision support systems

KEY POINTS

- Telemedicine intensive care units (tele-ICUs) cover more than 11% of ICU beds in the United States and produce enormous quantities of data, which can be used to create machine learning algorithms.
- Tele-ICU systems including clinical decision support systems have been shown to improve adherence to ICU best practices.
- Machine learning algorithms exist for sepsis detection, sepsis management, mechanical ventilation, false-alarm reduction, and ICU outcomes; validation using external data sets is important.
- Translating ICU machine learning algorithms to the tele-ICU requires the ability to generalize and adapt to a tele-ICU work flow that manages larger populations.

Disclosure: The Laboratory of Computational Physiology receives research funding from Philips Healthcare (United States). Dr O. Badawi is an employee of Philips Healthcare.
[a] Laboratory for Computational Physiology, Massachusetts Institute of Technology, Cambridge, MA, USA; [b] Department of Pulmonary, Critical Care, and Sleep Medicine, Beth Israel Deaconess Medical Center, Boston, MA, USA; [c] Patient Care Analytics, Philips Healthcare, Baltimore, MD, USA; [d] Department of Pharmacy Practice and Science, University of Maryland School of Pharmacy, Baltimore, MD, USA; [e] Department of Intensive Care, Wellington Hospital, Wellington, New Zealand
[1] Present address: E25-505, 77 Massachusetts Avenue, Cambridge, MA 02139.
[2] Present address: 217 East Redwood Street, Suite 1900, Baltimore, MD 21202.
* Corresponding author. Massachusetts Institute of Technology, E25-505, 77 Massachusetts Avenue, Cambridge, MA 02139.
E-mail address: lceli@mit.edu

Crit Care Clin 35 (2019) 483–495
https://doi.org/10.1016/j.ccc.2019.02.005
criticalcare.theclinics.com

INTRODUCTION

Over the last half-century, the telemedicine intensive care unit (tele-ICU) has grown from a daily video conference to a comprehensive high-bandwidth system connecting more than 11% of intensive care unit (ICU) beds in the United States to remote clinicians with real-time exchange and archiving of extensive patient data fed through algorithmic clinical decision support systems (CDSSs).[1,2] Machine learning (ML) has grown in parallel with the increasing availability of powerful computational resources. ML algorithms such as neural networks can process enormous quantities of data through multiple layers of features to elucidate novel interactions (**Fig. 1**). This article reviews the history of tele-ICU, examines the current state of ICU and tele-ICU CDSS (which can encompass predictive, detective, and prescriptive algorithms), and presents an overview of ML applications in the ICU that may be suitable for tele-ICU adaptation. In addition, it discusses issues to be considered when implementing tele-ICU CDSS, including staff perception and acceptance, human factors engineering, outcome measurement, and the need for rapid and continuous validation throughout the CDSS lifecycle. The development of clinically useful CDSS is not a simple task and its adaptation for the tele-ICU can be a formidable challenge, but the increasing accessibility of ML algorithms and large ICU databases for CDSS development and validation provides hope that a renaissance in tele-ICU CDSS may be coming soon.

HISTORY
Telemedicine Intensive Care Unit

The first implementation of tele-ICU care was in 1975, as a 2-way audiovisual link to provide remote intensivist consultations, with real-time data collected manually by consultants and outcomes obtained from a post hoc chart review.[1] The technology used did not make any provisions for the automatic acquisition, hardcopy transmission, or electronic storage of patient data. Furthermore, only 30% of the recommendations made by the remote intensivist were executed and the limited amount of time spent in direct communication with bedside physicians was considered a

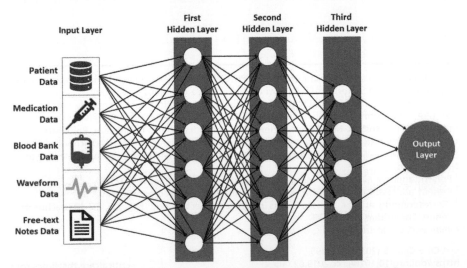

Fig. 1. Neural network example using readily available electronic medical data.

significant barrier to care.[3] These difficulties foreshadowed many of the challenges in developing effective tele-ICU CDSS.

By 1997, advancements in communications technology facilitated the deployment of a tele-ICU system capable of rapidly transmitting comprehensive patient data. Rosenfeld and colleagues[4] described a system providing access to real-time bedside monitor data, laboratory data, scanned hardcopy data (eg, electrocardiograms), daily video conferencing rounds with bedside physicians, twice-daily nursing discussions, and rapid bidirectional communication. Compared with 2 historical baseline periods, the implementation period had significantly lower severity-adjusted ICU mortality, severity-adjusted hospital mortality, ICU complication rate, and ICU length of stay (LOS).

It was evident at the time that these systems needed to incorporate tools that alleviate the cognitive burden on critical care providers. CDSS were developed using evidence-based clinical practice guidelines and protocols, disseminated using Web-based tools, and integrated into order entry systems.[5] Predictive alerts were developed to detect physiologic trends using vital signs and laboratory data before an overt clinical deterioration, allowing a small team of providers to monitor many patients. The clinical information system structured provider input, which was fused with the abundant clinical data generated during routine care to develop a data warehouse for future data mining and analysis.

As of 2014, continuous tele-ICU coverage was available for 11% of nonfederal hospital ICU beds for adults.[2] With tele-ICU coverage projected to grow a rate of 1% per year, it may have surpassed bedside intensivist coverage since then. Koninklijke Philips eICU, the successor to the Rosenfeld and colleagues'[4] system, is the predominant tele-ICU implementation in the United States, covering 99.2% of tele-ICU deployments based on Medicare data through 2010.[6]

Machine Learning in Critical Care

As the tele-ICU came of age, researchers developed novel uses for ML in critical care. Hart and Wyatt[7] assessed the ability of neural networks trained on 174 cases of chest pain to predict myocardial infarctions in a validation set of 73 cases, but found a false-negative rate of 27%. Doig and colleagues[8] developed a back-propagation associated-learning neural network using 27 features from 422 patients to model ICU mortality, but found it equivalent to logistic regression when used on training and validation sets. The investigators suggested larger data sets would allow prediction of ICU mortality with greater than 95% sensitivity and specificity. ML methods were applied in multiple other critical care contexts over the next 15 years with limited impact because of the small underlying data sets and lack of external reproducibility.

The last decade's advances in computing power and the availability of large clinical databases have allowed dramatic advancements in the application of ML to medicine. Ting and colleagues[9] described a deep learning system trained on 494,661 retinal images that accurately classifies diabetic retinopathy, possible glaucoma, and age-related diabetic retinopathy with an area under the receiver operating characteristic curve (AUROC) greater than 0.93 in all cases compared with professional graders. Moreover, external validation had an AUROC range of 0.889 to 0.983 using 10 additional data sets.

Electronic medical record (EMR) and tele-ICU adoption have exponentially increased the amount of digitally archived medical data. The large, rich, heterogeneous data sets that result have been used to develop novel clinical insights.[10,11] The deidentification of data sets has facilitated dissemination of data that were previously sequestered, such as the Medical Information Mart for Intensive Care database

(MIMIC-III)[12] and the eICU Collaborative Research Database (eICU-CRD).[13] The development of generalizable medical ML algorithms will only be possible using such large, comprehensive, heterogeneous, and granular data sets.

STATE OF CLINICAL DECISION SUPPORT SYSTEMS IN THE TELEMEDICINE INTENSIVE CARE UNIT

All tele-ICU outcome studies have been observational with predominantly pretest/posttest designs.[14,15] Tele-ICU implementations have differed significantly between studies and findings have been mixed. Highlighting the importance of effective implementation through clinical transformation, 2 major studies that failed to show significant benefit reflected poor cultural adoption: the tele-ICU team was prohibited from managing patients outside of code situations in approximately two-thirds of intervention patients.[16,17] Furthermore, studies have precluded analysis of the relative impact from individual factors in tele-ICU care, including CDSS.[18] Two studies met inclusion criteria for a systematic review, which found that tele-ICU care was associated with reductions in ICU mortality, hospital mortality, ICU LOS, and hospital LOS.[19]

In 2011, Lilly and colleagues[20] also found associations between tele-ICU care and increased adherence to best-practice guidelines (for prevention of venous thromboembolism [VTE], stress ulcers, cardiovascular complications, and ventilator-associated pneumonia) and lower risk of catheter-related bloodstream infection and ventilator-associated pneumonia. Lower tele-ICU mortalities persisted after adjusting for these differences, which were estimated to account for 25% of the hospital mortality and 30% of the ICU mortality declines. A 2014 multicenter pretest/posttest study further showed associations of tele-ICU care improvements in best-practice adherence and decreased mortality and LOS.[21]

It is reasonable to presume that CDSS deployment is a significant factor in improving best-practice adherence. Although the CDSS algorithms used in tele-ICU systems are proprietary, a number have been described in the literature. It is important to recognize that the work flow for tele-ICU clinicians is not identical to that of bedside staff, and therefore the design for tele-ICU CDSS may differ from bedside tools. Notably, a core feature of tele-ICU is population management, and many tools are designed to facilitate tele-ICU staff shifting roles as needed for a large population of ICU patients. Furthermore, no CDSS tool will improve outcomes without effective integration into work flow and a collaborative environment to support care at the bedside.

Patient Acuity

Williams and colleagues[22] described a 3-level color-coded acuity system for tele-ICU patients that incorporated time since ICU admission, vital sign stability, active titration and level of vasoactive agents, initiation of mechanical ventilation, emergent interventions, deescalation of therapies, safety concerns, and readiness for ICU transfer. The acuity category determined the frequency of tele-ICU nursing rounds and prioritized workflow. Other acuity scores for delirium, pain, and agitation evaluate ICU patients for corresponding factors related to screening, treatment, and adverse drug events, and present data in a dynamically changing dashboard for the population monitored.[23] However, the specific components are proprietary and not detailed in the tele-ICU literature.

Laboratory and Ordering Alerts

Tele-ICU deployments provided alerts for abnormal laboratory results before EMRs were widely used.[20] Medication dose adjustments can be prompted by creatinine clearance changes and computerized provider order entry can detect allergies and drug interactions.[5]

Best-practices Adherence

Routine monitoring of best practices based on clinical guidelines in domains such as VTE prophylaxis, stress ulcer prophylaxis, low tidal volume ventilation, β-blocker use, and glycemic control allows for real-time nonadherence notification and routine administrative auditing.[10] A retrospective multicenter study from 2009 to 2013 showed that adherence to best practices for VTE prophylaxis, low tidal volume ventilation, and glycemic control for tele-ICU patients significantly increased.[11] Remote screening with EMR prompting has been found to increase the likelihood of sedation interruption and spontaneous breathing trials, with an associated decrease in duration of mechanical ventilation, ICU LOS, and hospital LOS.[24] The rate of 3 hospital-associated infections did not differ despite remote screening for adherence to a ventilatory bundle and daily assessment of the need for central venous and urinary catheters.

Ventilator Management

Kalb and colleagues[25] studied the impact of tele-ICU–directed daily ventilator rounds in 11 hospitals with varying levels of ICU staffing. The rounds assessed adherence to low tidal volume ventilation but also addressed ventilator settings, sedation strategies, spontaneous breathing trials, and readiness for ventilator liberation. The intervention was associated with significant increase in low tidal volume ventilation adherence, from 29.5% before implementation to 44.9% after 9 months, and the improvement persisted 6 months later (52.0%). There was also an associated improvement in the Acute Physiology and Chronic Health Evaluation IV (APACHE-IV)–adjusted ICU mortality ratio (0.94 vs 0.67 after 9 months).

Sepsis Screening and Management

Rincon and colleagues[26] described the implementation of a tele-ICU nurse–driven program to facilitate early identification of patients with severe sepsis and prompt initiation of bundled care based on what were considered best practices at the time. From 2006 to 2008 the tele-ICU nurses manually performed 89,921 screens between 10 hospitals and identified 5437 patients with severe sepsis. Screening was associated with increases in timely antibiotic administration (74% vs 55%), serum lactate measurement (66% vs 50%), 20 mL/kg fluid bolus administration (70% vs 23%), and central line placement (50% vs 33%). The evolving definition of sepsis and its standard of care over the last several years exemplify a common issue in developing robust CDSS tools with validation for syndromes that are not firmly defined.[27]

Automated sepsis screens with 90% sensitivity and 80% specificity have reduced the burden of manually screening patients but still have a low positive predictive value because of the small population at risk.[27] Randomized controlled trials of automated sepsis monitoring systems in a single academic tertiary care center without tele-ICU found no significant differences in median time to new antibiotics, fluid administration, time to completion of a sepsis bundle or individual elements, ventilator-free days, ICU-free days, ICU LOS, hospital LOS, ICU mortality, and in-hospital mortality.[28,29] Nevertheless, automated sepsis screening remains an area of active research and development in the tele-ICU.[30]

Physiologic Instability Alerts

The proprietary algorithms implemented by tele-ICU providers have not been described in detail in the published literature. However, they claim the ability to detect early signs of physiologic instability and notify providers.[21] An association between shorter alarm response times and shorter ICU LOS was found based on observational data.[21] However, use of a tele-ICU model does not guarantee a timely response to physiologic instability alarms.[31]

Intensive Care Unit Readmission Risk

McShea and colleagues[32] reported the development of an initial retrospective exploratory cohort using 123,848 ICU stays between 2005 and 2007 from the Philips eResearch Institute (eRI) database to create a model predicting death or ICU readmission within 48 hours of ICU discharge. The logistic regression model was found to have a c-index predicting death of 0.89 and ICU readmission of 0.61.

Subsequently, Badawi and Breslow[33] described the development and internal validation of a different multivariable logistic regression model predicting death or ICU readmission within 48 hours of ICU discharge. The retrospective cohort was also derived from the eRI database taking 704,963 patients meeting inclusion criteria at 219 hospitals between 2007 and 2011, with 2:1 allocation to the development and validation. Of the initial 59 variables considered, the final model included 26 for death and 23 for ICU readmission, 8 of which were known at the time of admission. The readmission model had a median AUROC of 0.71, whereas the mortality prediction model had a median AUROC of 0.92; both performed similarly in the development set and validation set. Compared with prior studies that used a single outcome, separating the models for readmission and death resulted in better performance.

Badawi and colleagues'[34] models were the basis for the Philips eICU Discharge Readiness Score (DRS), which was later compared with other ICU severity of illness scores. The eRI database was used to develop a new cohort of 561,478 patients meeting inclusion criteria at 208 hospitals from 2013 to 2016. The DRS, APACHE-IV score, and Sequential Organ Failure Assessment (SOFA) score were calculated hourly from the fourth hour of ICU admission. The DRS showed higher discrimination for ICU mortality (AUROC, 0.942) than the APACHE-IV score (AUROC, 0.895) and the SOFA score (AUROC, 0.862). Some of the discrepancies were hypothesized to be partially related to increasing APACHE-IV and SOFA scores in those who survive caused by the inclusion of the worst value over the prior 24 hours, compared with DRS's inclusion of more recent values reflecting improvement in the clinical condition.

FUTURE TELEMEDICINE INTENSIVE CARE UNIT APPLICATIONS OF MACHINE LEARNING

The intersection of so-called big data and clinical decision support has provided an opportunity for advancements in the creation of and ability to generalize models. The existing tele-ICU clinical decision support models were generated using classic logistic regression techniques,[33] but novel ML algorithms are being developed from larger and richer data sets to address a wide variety of clinical dilemmas in critical care (**Table 1**).[35,36] External validation of these efforts using widely available data sets such as MIMIC-III[12] and eICU-CRD[13] will help guide the application of ML to the tele-ICU going forward.

Although predictive models are often a focus of research, any model predicting a rare outcome will have a low positive predictive value even if the discrimination is very high. An overlooked fact in designing and evaluating CDSS is that the target should only be the unrecognized prevalence of a condition rather than the total prevalence as the tool will only be useful in predicting what is not already known to the

Table 1 Recent studies of machine learning applicable to critical care	
Sepsis	• Numerous studies evaluating a variety of ML methods to predict sepsis 3–12 h before onset[37–42] • Nonblinded randomized controlled trial of a proprietary ML algorithm (vs EMR severe sepsis alert) showed shorter ICU and hospital LOS and lower in-hospital mortality[43] • Retrospective study of ICU complications before and after implementation of real-time predictive analytics monitoring display associated with decrease in sepsis incidence[44] • Reinforcement learning model developed to assess optimal treatment of patients with septic shock (vasopressors vs IV fluids) predicted higher-value treatments than clinicians[45] • Switching-state autoregressive model predicted vasopressor administration and successful vasopressor weaning[46]
Mechanical Ventilation	• Random forest algorithm showed significant agreement with clinical experts in detecting ventilator asynchrony[51] • Multiple ML algorithms identified ventilator dyssynchrony, but the best-performing model differed by type of event[52] • Gradient-boosted decision trees algorithm predicted need for prolonged mechanical ventilation (AUROC, 0.820) and tracheostomy (AUROC, 0.830) at time of ICU admission[53] • Support vector machine algorithm trained using heart rate variability and patient-specific calibration data discriminated between light and deep sedation with 75% accuracy[54]
False-alarm Reduction	• Random forest model trained on human annotated alerts discriminated between true and false alarms for peripheral oximetry, blood pressure, and respiratory rate[55] • Multiple ML algorithms were used by teams competing to classify true and false arrhythmia alarms[56]
ICU Outcomes	• Gradient-boosting decision tree model developed using a single-center 14,962-patient cohort to predict the risk of ICU readmission was superior to other risk assessments (AUROC, 0.76 vs 0.58–0.65); validation in MIMIC-III had comparable results (AUROC, 0.71 vs 0.57–0.58)[57] • Random forest model developed using a single-center 6376-patient cohort to predict hospital-acquired pressure injury had an AUROC of 0.79 for stage 1 and stage 2+ injuries[58] • Recurrent neural network models developed using a single-center 9269-cardiac surgery patient cohort to predict mortality, renal replacement therapy, and postoperative bleeding requiring surgery outperformed other predictors in all outcomes (AUROCs of 0.95 vs 0.71, 0.96 vs 0.72, and 0.87 vs 0.53 respectively). Validation in MIMIC-III had comparable results[59] • Unstructured text data added to ML models from MIMIC-III improved prediction of death or prolonged ICU stay. Gradient-boosted machines slightly outperformed random forests, elastic net regression, and logistic regression[60] • Gradient-boosted decision tree model developed using a 53-center 237,173-patient ICU cohort predicted in-hospital mortality well (AUROC, 0.951 in training subset and 0.943 in validation subset)[61]

user.[27] One option to address this challenge is by diverting the low-yield but important screening activity to tele-ICU staff, allowing bedside staff to remain focused on their clinical activities. The following areas are some that the authors consider to be exciting and promising avenues potentially applicable in the tele-ICU.

Sepsis Prediction

Many ML algorithms to predict sepsis from clinical data have been developed:

- An elastic net logistic classifier applied to a single-center 1110-patient cohort to predict sepsis 4 hours before onset found that high-resolution vital signs combined with sociodemographic and clinical characteristics achieved an AUROC of 0.78.[37]
- Coupled hidden Markov models were compared with nonlinear support vector machine models applied to a single-center 1310-patient cohort from a MIMIC-III predecessor to predict septic shock during sepsis.[38]
- InSight, a proprietary ML model to predict sepsis 3 hours before onset developed from a MIMIC-III predecessor,[39] was then validated using the larger MIMIC-III cohort and found to outperform other assessments of sepsis (eg, SOFA scores) with an AUROC of 0.880 and to still perform well when tested with randomly missing data.[40]
- Deep learning models incorporating feedforward neural networks and long short-term memory to predict sepsis 3 hours before onset were derived using a 5803-patient cohort from a MIMIC-III predecessor and found to be capable of unsupervised feature extraction with improved performance compared with a proprietary regression model using hand-crafted features.[41]

More recently, ML approaches to sepsis detection have been validated in external data sets and real-world applications. Nemati and colleagues[42] developed a modified Weibull-Cox proportional hazards 65-feature model to predict sepsis 4 to 12 hours before onset using an internal 2-center 27,527-patient cohort with an AUROC of 0.83 to 0.85 and validated it using a 42,411-patient cohort from MIMIC-III with similar results (AUROC, 0.79–0.84). Using a larger data set than earlier models allowed prediction over significantly longer periods.

Shimabukuro and colleagues[43] performed the first randomized controlled trial of ML algorithms for sepsis detection in 2016. Although the InSight algorithm used 9 vital signs during its development,[39] the data requirements are flexible and had previously been evaluated using alternatives.[40] Shimabukuro and colleagues'[43] model included 6 features (age, blood pressure, heart rate, temperature, respiratory rate, and peripheral oxygen saturation) measured hourly in the 142 patients randomized during the 3-month study. Compared with a group monitored by the preexisting EMR severe sepsis alert system, the group monitored by the ML algorithm had significantly lower hospital LOS (10.3 days vs 13.0 days; $P = .042$), ICU LOS (6.31 days vs 8.40 days; $P = .030$), and in-hospital mortality (8.96% vs 21.3%; $P = .018$).[43] Note that caution must be taken in generalizing findings from a small, single-center, nonblinded trial; however, other studies have shown benefits from continuous real-time monitoring with multivariate predictive models for septic shock.[44]

Sepsis Management

Komorowski and colleagues[45] used a reinforcement learning agent to develop an artificial intelligence (AI) policy assessing whether vasopressors or intravenous (IV) fluids are the optimal intervention for a given patient with septic shock. The model was developed using a single-center 17,083-patient cohort from MIMIC-III, tested using a 128-center 79,073-patient cohort from the eRI database, and included 48 variables coded as a time-series over a 72-hour period around the estimated time of sepsis onset. A Markov decision process (MDP) modeled transitions between 750 discrete mutually exclusive patient states identified on cluster analysis. The theoretic optimum policy identified decisions (limited to actions taken by the clinician in the data set) that maximized rewards (ie, survival) for solving the MDP.

Bootstrapping evaluation of 500 candidate models and 500 clustering solutions on the MIMIC-III validation cohort provided the optimal model to be tested against the eRI database. The AI policy recommended higher vasopressor doses and lower IV fluid doses on average. Vasopressors were administered in 17% of eRI patients, whereas the AI policy recommended vasopressors in 30%. Mortality was shown to increase in a dose-dependent fashion as clinician intervention doses diverged from the AI policy recommendations.[45] An earlier study showed that a switching-state autoregressive model can predict vasopressor administration and weaning.[46]

Mechanical Ventilation

Lung protective ventilation decreases mortality in acute respiratory distress syndrome, and other causes of respiratory failure,[47,48] but the root cause of the difference is unclear.[49,50] The ability of modern mechanical ventilators to generate breath-to-breath pressure-volume curves offers unique opportunities to create rich high-bandwidth data sets. ML applied to a data set combining waveform and EMR data could detect factors affecting patient outcomes and optimize individual ventilator management.

A random forest model was able to discriminate between ventilator waveforms showing no asynchrony, delayed termination, and premature termination to a similar degree as clinical experts (kappa coefficients, 0.90, 0.90, and 0.91 respectively).[51] ML algorithms have also been applied to identify ventilator dyssynchrony from waveforms, and found to be effective at identifying double-triggered breaths, flow-limited breaths, and synchronous breaths, although the best model varied by dyssynchrony (AUROC, 0.89–0.95).[52]

TELEMEDICINE INTENSIVE CARE UNIT CLINICAL DECISION SUPPORT SYSTEM CONSIDERATIONS

There is abundant research on factors affecting bedside staff perception and acceptance of tele-ICU. Staff appreciate if tele-ICU provides improved workflow, improved monitoring, rapid availability, specialty expertise, and staff familiarity, but issues of unrealistic expectations and poor communication were barriers.[62–65] More recently Kahn and colleagues[66] found that tele-ICU systems perceived to be "appropriate, responsive, consistent, and integrated with bedside workflows" were associated with decreased mortality after being deployed. Tele-ICU CDSS must achieve these goals in addition to being autonomous, generalizable, transparent, coherent, and ideally educational; a black box is not an adequate decision aide.

These factors must be the foundation of tele-ICU ML CDSS development going forward. Tele-ICU nurses have been reported to care for 30 to 52 patients simultaneously,[67] with a median of 3 nurses per tele-ICU hub.[31] As the number of CDSS algorithms proliferate, they must be integrated into the tele-ICU workflow, which will differ significantly from the bedside because of the population-level surveillance taking place. Human factors engineering may be needed to ensure that CDSS that is effective at the bedside is not a burden in the tele-ICU.[30] CDSS deployment should be studied routinely using outcomes in both the short term (eg, best-practice adherence) and long term (eg, mortality). Furthermore, the constantly evolving state of the art in medicine requires rapid validation of CDSS models using large data sets as well as ongoing reevaluation and recalibration as circumstances change. Creating tele-ICU

ML CDSS will be challenging but has the potential to provide greater impact for more patients than any single-center CDSS.

SUMMARY

The use of ML in critical care CDSS is a rapidly developing field. The availability of large, comprehensive, granular data sets is fueling growth in ML algorithms that will be far more accurate and generalizable than in years past. The tele-ICU provides a framework to deploy ML algorithms at scale but will require emphasis on usability for monitoring large patient populations and studies of their effects on patient outcomes.

REFERENCES

1. Grundy BL, Crawford P, Jones PK, et al. Telemedicine in critical care: an experiment in health care delivery. JACEP 1977;6(10):439–44.
2. Lilly CM, Zubrow MT, Kempner KM, et al. Critical care telemedicine: evolution and state of the art. Crit Care Med 2014;42(11):2429–36.
3. Grundy BL, Jones PK, Lovitt A. Telemedicine in critical care: problems in design, implementation, and assessment. Crit Care Med 1982;10(7):471–5.
4. Rosenfeld BA, Dorman T, Breslow MJ, et al. Intensive care unit telemedicine: alternate paradigm for providing continuous intensivist care. Crit Care Med 2000;28(12):3925–31.
5. Celi LA, Hassan E, Marquardt C, et al. The eICU: it's not just telemedicine. Crit Care Med 2001;29(8 Suppl):N183–9.
6. Kahn JM, Le TQ, Barnato AE, et al. ICU telemedicine and critical care mortality: a national effectiveness study. Med Care 2016;54(3):319–25.
7. Hart A, Wyatt J. Connectionist models in medicine: an investigation of their potential. In: Hunter J, Cookson J, Wyatt J, editors. AIME 89. Lecture notes in medical informatics. Berlin: Springer; 1989. p. 115–24.
8. Doig GS, Inman KJ, Sibbald WJ, et al. Modeling mortality in the intensive care unit: comparing the performance of a back-propagation, associative-learning neural network with multivariate logistic regression. Proc Annu Symp Comput Appl Med Care 1993;361–5.
9. Ting DSW, Cheung CY-L, Lim G, et al. Development and validation of a deep learning system for diabetic retinopathy and related eye diseases using retinal images from multiethnic populations with diabetes. JAMA 2017;318(22):2211–23.
10. Lilly CM, Zuckerman IH, Badawi O, et al. Benchmark data from more than 240,000 adults that reflect the current practice of critical care in the United States. Chest 2011;140(5):1232–42.
11. Lilly CM, Swami S, Liu X, et al. Five-year trends of critical care practice and outcomes. Chest 2017;152(4):723–35.
12. Johnson AEW, Pollard TJ, Shen L, et al. MIMIC-III, a freely accessible critical care database. Sci Data 2016;3:160035.
13. Pollard TJ, Johnson AEW, Raffa JD, et al. The eICU Collaborative Research Database, a freely available multi-center database for critical care research. Sci Data 2018;5:180178.
14. Venkataraman R, Ramakrishnan N. Outcomes related to telemedicine in the intensive care unit: what we know and would like to know. Crit Care Clin 2015;31(2):225–37.

15. Vranas KC, Slatore CG, Kerlin MP. Telemedicine coverage of intensive care units: a narrative review. Ann Am Thorac Soc 2018. https://doi.org/10.1513/AnnalsATS. 201804-225FR.

16. Morrison JL, Cai Q, Davis N, et al. Clinical and economic outcomes of the electronic intensive care unit: results from two community hospitals. Crit Care Med 2010;38(1):2–8.

17. Thomas EJ, Lucke JF, Wueste L, et al. Association of telemedicine for remote monitoring of intensive care patients with mortality, complications, and length of stay. JAMA 2009;302(24):2671–8.

18. Kahn JM, Hill NS, Lilly CM, et al. The research agenda in ICU telemedicine: a statement from the Critical Care Societies Collaborative. Chest 2011;140(1): 230–8.

19. Mackintosh N, Terblanche M, Maharaj R, et al. Telemedicine with clinical decision support for critical care: a systematic review. Syst Rev 2016;5(1):176.

20. Lilly CM, Cody S, Zhao H, et al. Hospital mortality, length of stay, and preventable complications among critically ill patients before and after tele-ICU reengineering of critical care processes. JAMA 2011;305(21):2175–83.

21. Lilly CM, McLaughlin JM, Zhao H, et al. A multicenter study of ICU telemedicine reengineering of adult critical care. Chest 2014;145(3):500–7.

22. Williams L-M, Hubbard KE, Daye O, et al. Telenursing in the intensive care unit: transforming nursing practice. Crit Care Nurse 2012;32(6):62–9.

23. Philips eICU Research Institute (eRI). Philips. Available at: https://www.usa. philips.com/healthcare/solutions/enterprise-telehealth/eri. Accessed November 9, 2018.

24. Kahn JM, Gunn SR, Lorenz HL, et al. Impact of nurse-led remote screening and prompting for evidence-based practices in the ICU*. Crit Care Med 2014;42(4): 896–904.

25. Kalb T, Raikhelkar J, Meyer S, et al. A multicenter population-based effectiveness study of teleintensive care unit-directed ventilator rounds demonstrating improved adherence to a protective lung strategy, decreased ventilator duration, and decreased intensive care unit mortality. J Crit Care 2014;29(4):691.e7-14.

26. Rincon TA, Bourke G, Seiver A. Standardizing sepsis screening and management via a tele-ICU program improves patient care. Telemed J E Health 2011;17(7): 560–4.

27. Badawi O, Hassan E. Telemedicine and the patient with sepsis. Crit Care Clin 2015;31(2):291–304.

28. Hooper MH, Weavind L, Wheeler AP, et al. Randomized trial of automated, electronic monitoring to facilitate early detection of sepsis in the intensive care unit*. Crit Care Med 2012;40(7):2096–101.

29. Semler MW, Weavind L, Hooper MH, et al. An electronic tool for the evaluation and treatment of sepsis in the ICU: a randomized controlled trial. Crit Care Med 2015;43(8):1595–602.

30. Rincon TA, Manos EL, Pierce JD. Telehealth intensive care unit nurse surveillance of sepsis. Comput Inform Nurs 2017;35(9):459–64.

31. Lilly CM, Fisher KA, Ries M, et al. A national ICU telemedicine survey: validation and results. Chest 2012;142(1):40–7.

32. McShea M, Holl R, Badawi O, et al. The eICU research institute - a collaboration between industry, health-care providers, and academia. IEEE Eng Med Biol Mag 2010;29(2):18–25.

33. Badawi O, Breslow MJ. Readmissions and death after ICU discharge: development and validation of two predictive models. PLoS One 2012;7(11):e48758.

34. Badawi O, Liu X, Hassan E, et al. Evaluation of ICU risk models adapted for use as continuous markers of severity of illness throughout the ICU stay. Crit Care Med 2018;46(3):361–7.

35. Rush B, Celi LA, Stone DJ. Applying machine learning to continuously monitored physiological data. J Clin Monit Comput 2018. https://doi.org/10.1007/s10877-018-0219-z.

36. Sanchez-Pinto LN, Luo Y, Churpek MM. Big data and data science in critical care. Chest 2018. https://doi.org/10.1016/j.chest.2018.04.037.

37. Shashikumar SP, Stanley MD, Sadiq I, et al. Early sepsis detection in critical care patients using multiscale blood pressure and heart rate dynamics. J Electrocardiol 2017;50(6):739–43.

38. Ghosh S, Li J, Cao L, et al. Septic shock prediction for ICU patients via coupled HMM walking on sequential contrast patterns. J Biomed Inform 2017;66:19–31.

39. Calvert JS, Price DA, Chettipally UK, et al. A computational approach to early sepsis detection. Comput Biol Med 2016;74:69–73.

40. Desautels T, Calvert J, Hoffman J, et al. Prediction of sepsis in the intensive care unit with minimal electronic health record data: a machine learning approach. JMIR Med Inform 2016;4(3):e28.

41. Kam HJ, Kim HY. Learning representations for the early detection of sepsis with deep neural networks. Comput Biol Med 2017;89:248–55.

42. Nemati S, Holder A, Razmi F, et al. An interpretable machine learning model for accurate prediction of sepsis in the ICU. Crit Care Med 2018;46(4):547–53.

43. Shimabukuro DW, Barton CW, Feldman MD, et al. Effect of a machine learning-based severe sepsis prediction algorithm on patient survival and hospital length of stay: a randomised clinical trial. BMJ Open Respir Res 2017;4(1):e000234.

44. Ruminski CM, Clark MT, Lake DE, et al. Impact of predictive analytics based on continuous cardiorespiratory monitoring in a surgical and trauma intensive care unit. J Clin Monit Comput 2018. https://doi.org/10.1007/s10877-018-0194-4.

45. Komorowski M, Celi LA, Badawi O, et al. The Artificial Intelligence Clinician learns optimal treatment strategies for sepsis in intensive care. Nat Med 2018. https://doi.org/10.1038/s41591-018-0213-5.

46. Wu M, Ghassemi M, Feng M, et al. Understanding vasopressor intervention and weaning: risk prediction in a public heterogeneous clinical time series database. J Am Med Inform Assoc 2017;24(3):488–95.

47. Acute Respiratory Distress Syndrome Network, Brower RG, Matthay MA, Morris A, et al. Ventilation with lower tidal volumes as compared with traditional tidal volumes for acute lung injury and the acute respiratory distress syndrome. N Engl J Med 2000;342(18):1301–8.

48. Serpa Neto A, Cardoso SO, Manetta JA, et al. Association between use of lung-protective ventilation with lower tidal volumes and clinical outcomes among patients without acute respiratory distress syndrome: a meta-analysis. JAMA 2012;308(16):1651–9.

49. Amato MBP, Meade MO, Slutsky AS, et al. Driving pressure and survival in the acute respiratory distress syndrome. N Engl J Med 2015;372(8):747–55.

50. Serpa Neto A, Deliberato RO, Johnson AEW, et al. Mechanical power of ventilation is associated with mortality in critically ill patients: an analysis of patients in two observational cohorts. Intensive Care Med 2018. https://doi.org/10.1007/s00134-018-5375-6.

51. Gholami B, Phan TS, Haddad WM, et al. Replicating human expertise of mechanical ventilation waveform analysis in detecting patient-ventilator cycling asynchrony using machine learning. Comput Biol Med 2018;97:137–44.

52. Sottile PD, Albers D, Higgins C, et al. The association between ventilator dyssynchrony, delivered tidal volume, and sedation using a novel automated ventilator dyssynchrony detection algorithm. Crit Care Med 2018;46(2):e151–7.
53. Parreco J, Hidalgo A, Parks JJ, et al. Using artificial intelligence to predict prolonged mechanical ventilation and tracheostomy placement. J Surg Res 2018; 228:179–87.
54. Nagaraj SB, Biswal S, Boyle EJ, et al. Patient-specific classification of ICU sedation levels from heart rate variability. Crit Care Med 2017;45(7):e683–90.
55. Chen L, Dubrawski A, Wang D, et al. Using supervised machine learning to classify real alerts and artifact in online multisignal vital sign monitoring data. Crit Care Med 2016;44(7):e456–63.
56. Clifford GD, Silva I, Moody B, et al. False alarm reduction in critical care. Physiol Meas 2016;37(8):E5–23.
57. Rojas JC, Carey KA, Edelson DP, et al. Predicting intensive care unit readmission with machine learning using electronic health record data. Ann Am Thorac Soc 2018;15(7):846–53.
58. Alderden J, Pepper GA, Wilson A, et al. Predicting pressure injury in critical care patients: a machine-learning model. Am J Crit Care 2018;27(6):461–8.
59. Meyer A, Zverinski D, Pfahringer B, et al. Machine learning for real-time prediction of complications in critical care: a retrospective study. Lancet Respir Med 2018. https://doi.org/10.1016/S2213-2600(18)30300-X.
60. Weissman GE, Hubbard RA, Ungar LH, et al. Inclusion of unstructured clinical text improves early prediction of death or prolonged ICU stay. Crit Care Med 2018;46(7):1125–32.
61. Delahanty RJ, Kaufman D, Jones SS. Development and evaluation of an automated machine learning algorithm for in-hospital mortality risk adjustment among critical care patients. Crit Care Med 2018;46(6):e481–8.
62. Kleinpell R, Barden C, Rincon T, et al. Assessing the impact of telemedicine on nursing care in intensive care units. Am J Crit Care 2016;25(1):e14–20.
63. Wilkes MS, Marcin JP, Ritter LA, et al. Organizational and teamwork factors of tele-intensive care units. Am J Crit Care 2016;25(5):431–9.
64. Goedken CC, Moeckli J, Cram PM, et al. Introduction of Tele-ICU in rural hospitals: changing organisational culture to harness benefits. Intensive Crit Care Nurs 2017;40:51–6.
65. Thomas JT, Moeckli J, Mengeling MA, et al. Bedside critical care staff use of intensive care unit telemedicine: comparisons by intensive care unit complexity. Telemed J E Health 2017;23(9):718–25.
66. Kahn JM, Rak KJ, Kuza CC, et al. Determinants of intensive care unit telemedicine effectiveness: an ethnographic study. Am J Respir Crit Care Med 2018. https://doi.org/10.1164/rccm.201802-0259OC.
67. Hoonakker PLT, Pecanac KE, Brown RL, et al. Virtual collaboration, satisfaction, and trust between nurses in the tele-ICU and ICUs: results of a multilevel analysis. J Crit Care 2017;37:224–9.

Intensive Care Unit Telemedicine

Innovations and Limitations

William Bender, MD, MPH[a],
Cheryl A. Hiddleson, MSN, RN, CENP, CCRN-E[b],
Timothy G. Buchman, PhD, MD, MCCM[c],*

KEYWORDS

- Innovation • Limitation • Telemedicine • Intensive care unit

KEY POINTS

- Intensive care unit (ICU) telemedicine denotes an established tool that can help alleviate some of the issues faced by the field of critical care while also serving as a springboard for innovative improvements in the future.
- ICU telemedicine programs have proven to be an effective solution for delivering ICU care in resource-limited environments and in the face of intensivist staffing shortfalls.
- The inclusion of advanced practice providers, more formal inclusion in medical education, and concurrent utilization of machine learning technologies represent future areas of expansion for ICU telemedicine.
- The computational infrastructure of ICU telemedicine promises robust globalization of critical care services.

INTRODUCTION

The demands of critical care continue to grow, fueled by the aging population (and the aging population's disproportionate needs related to chronic medical conditions), by the maldistribution of intensive care resources, by the slow supply of appropriately trained new providers, and by retirement and death of aged providers. The growing demand has been identified by critical care providers and their associated professional societies.[1–4] The delivery of critical care requires considerable investment from a resource perspective and a financial one. In a 10-year period from 2000 until

---

Disclosure Statement: The authors have nothing to disclose.
[a] Division of Pulmonary, Allergy, Critical Care and Sleep Medicine, Emory University School of Medicine, 5673 Peachtree Dunwoody Road, Suite 502, Atlanta, GA 30342, USA; [b] Emory eICU Center, Emory Healthcare Incorporated, 5671 Peachtree Dunwoody Road, Suite 275, Atlanta, GA 30342, USA; [c] Emory University School of Medicine, 1440 Clifton Road Northeast, Suite 313, Atlanta, GA 30322, USA
* Corresponding author.
E-mail address: tbuchma@emory.edu

Crit Care Clin 35 (2019) 497–509
https://doi.org/10.1016/j.ccc.2019.02.011
0749-0704/19/© 2019 Elsevier Inc. All rights reserved.

2010, the cost for the provision of critical care to Medicare and Medicaid beneficiaries nearly doubled to just over $100 billion, while accounting for nearly 1% of the US gross domestic product.[5] It is not surprising then that critical care has been the target of numerous attempts to optimize efficiency, effectiveness, and quality.

Intensive care unit (ICU) telemedicine, defined as the remote provision of critical care facilitated by audiovisual conferencing technology, represents 1 strategy to improve efficiency and reduce cost.[6] ICU telemedicine implementations have continued to grow, with approximately 20% of adult ICU beds in the United States currently supported. ICU telemedicine has been associated with successful outcomes, including decreased costs and reduced malpractice claims.[7,8] The implementation models fall into 3 general classes:

Centralized telehealth, where care services originate from a centralized hub and are then delivered out to remote facilities

Decentralized telehealth, which represents more of a process given that there is no established monitoring facility or staff but rather a connected collection of computers and mobile devices often established at sites of convenience

Redisplay/support systems, which allow for collection and analysis of varying types of patient-generated clinical data[9–13]

Leveraging telecommunications technology for the delivery of critical care has not only allowed for novel solutions to issues faced by the field, but also has set the stage for a number of potential innovative enhancements in the future.

RECENT INNOVATIONS IN INTENSIVE CARE UNIT TELEMEDICINE
Critical Care Provider Shortage

The alarm around critical care provider staffing shortages was raised in 2000 in a study commissioned and reported by the Committee on Manpower for Pulmonary and Critical Care Societies, which represented a combined effort from members of the American Thoracic Society, the American College of Chest Physicians, and the Society of Critical Care Medicine. The report foresaw an unrelenting increase in demand for care coupled with a stagnant supply of intensivists, resulting in projections of intensivist hours meeting only 22% of demand by 2020 and 35% of demand by 2030.[2] That report also served as the impetus for the Framing Options for Critical Care in the United States (FOCCUS) report, which was crafted to address strategies to recruit and sustain an adequate critical care workforce.

There are similar supply and demand challenges forecast for critical care nurses. There is a predicted increase of 26% in demand for acute and critical care nurses in the United States from 2010 to 2024. The demand will not be met. Although the shortfall is partially attributable to the care requirements of an aging population and the retirement of large numbers of similarly aging nurses, it is compounded by 2 pipeline problems. One problem relates to insufficient numbers of qualified faculty to teach in accredited nursing schools; more than 60,000 otherwise acceptable candidates are turned away annually.[14] The second problem relates to insufficient graduate training slots; many hospitals hire only experienced nurses into critical care units, leaving new graduates with few options for employment.[15]

FOCCUS included discussion about information technology as a tool to combat this issue, and the authors specifically noted that "continuous remote intensivist staffing with video conferencing and computer-based data transmission may reduce ICU and hospital mortality, ICU complications, and ICU and hospital length of stay and costs. If supported by subsequent studies, the combination of informatics and telemedicine could promote more effective use of intensivists and promote quality, particularly in remote regions."[16] Rosenfeld and colleagues had already reported on experience with around-the-clock remote ICU management of patients in an ICU without continuous presence of an (on-site) intensivist. This observational study was conducted with 2 retrospective baseline periods along with a prospective intervention period in a 450-bed academic-affiliated hospital. During the intervention period, the remote intensivist provided 24-hour monitoring of all the ICU patients via video conferencing, along with transmission and near real-time display of patient care data normally available only at the bedside.[17] The telemedicine intervention was associated with a number of significant improvements, including a reduction in severity-adjusted ICU mortality in the hospital mortality. ICU length of stay declined by 34% and 30% (when compared with both baseline periods), and overall ICU costs decreased by 33% and 36%; additionally, there was a concomitant decrease in the incidence of complications.[17]

Subsequent investigations have continued to suggest that ICU telemedicine is an effective strategy for handling increased ICU staffing needs with associated improvements in quality. Reports emerged from various care environments including that of rural and urban hospitals, as well as community and academic medical centers. Given that over one-third of all US hospitals are rural, Zawada and colleagues examined the effects of the implementation of an ICU telemedicine system across the upper Midwest in the United States.[18–20] This program consisted of around-the-clock staffing of a remote care center by 1 critical care nurse and clerical support person along with 20 hours per day staffing by a critical care physician. The remote teams supported 1 tertiary referral hospital (with a 2- bed mixed medical and surgical ICU without dedicated intensivist staffing), 3 rural regional hospitals (with 10, 6, and 10 ICU beds, respectively), 2 community hospitals (with <100 beds total), and 9 critical access hospitals (<25 beds total). This program was associated with significant reductions in ICU mortality, ICU length of stay, hospital mortality, and hospital length of stay.[19,20] In addition, satisfaction and acceptance of the program were high across all of the participating sites.[19]

Lilly and colleagues examined the association of a telemedicine ICU intervention with hospital mortality, length of stay, and the presence of preventable complications in an academic medical center. This prospective, unblinded, stepped wedge study reported significant reductions in ICU mortality, ICU length of stay, hospital mortality, and hospital length of stay.[21] Significantly higher rates of best clinical practice adherence were attributed to the tele-ICU intervention, including protocols aimed at the prevention of deep vein thrombosis, stress ulcer prophylaxis, and ventilator-associated pneumonia. Interestingly, improvement for the tele-ICU intervention seemed greater for patients admitted after 8 p.m. During the preintervention period, these overnight admissions were reviewed only by telephone by the attending physician at the discretion of the bedside (either house staff or affiliate provider) team. During the intervention period, these overnight admissions were directly assessed by the tele-ICU team with plans of care then being developed and shared with the bedside providers.[21]

A recent meta-analysis examined the effect of ICU telemedicine implementation on ICU mortality.[22] Associated subgroup differences among ICUs with high and low baseline observed-to-predicted mortality ratios were also studied. Implementation was associated with an overall reduction in ICU mortality. In addition, for ICUs with high observed-to-predicted mortality ratios (>1), the introduction of ICU telemedicine was also significantly associated with a reduction in mortality. This relationship did not exist in ICUs with low (<1) baseline observed-to-predicted mortality ratios.[22]

Emory Healthcare gained similar improvements with the initiation of telemedicine ICU coverage. This health care system consists of several tertiary hospitals, each with a variety of subspecialty critical care capabilities, spread across the metropolitan Atlanta area. Emory's eICU Center provides support to 5 hospitals, including 158 ICU beds and mobile carts or in-room systems that allow for ICU without walls support to emergency departments. One of the hospitals served is a rural hospital that is not part of Emory Healthcare. The eICU Center uses an interprofessional and collaborative model of care that emphasizes a pivotal safety officer role for critical care nurses behind the camera who identify and assess threats and then assign tasks either to the eICU physician or to the bedside staff.[1] The Emory critical care model emphasizes advanced practice providers (APPs) at the bedside. The introduction of remote expert nurses and physicians to support APPs in a suburban tertiary hospital making the transition from community- to academic-centered practice resulted in marked and sustained improvements in ICU mortality and hospital length of stay (**Fig. 1**). The authors' local experience suggests that ICU telemedicine roles may be attractive to seasoned critical care physicians and nurses on the cusp of retirement. The physical demands and emotional stresses are perceived to be diminished compared with those experienced at the bedside.

Developing Countries and Resource-Limited Situations

Although ICU telemedicine has continued with increased growth and acceptance within the United States and in the Middle East and Japan, it has also recently begun to gain traction in more resource-limited areas.[23,24] The developing world, natural disasters, and combat environments are increasingly being explored as avenues by which telemedicine can be further utilized. Given that these settings tend to have higher associated levels of morbidity and mortality and also lack the presence of sustained, effective infrastructure along with consistent, appropriate skill sets, it is understandable why they are attractive targets for the specific implementation of ICU telemedicine services.

Critinext represents Asia's first tele-ICU system, and it currently provides coverage to 350 ICU beds in 10 different cities in India.[25,26] Implementation has helped guide the initiation of renal replacement therapy in critically ill patients and has also been associated with improved mortality along with decreased frequency of catheter-associated bloodstream infections.[27,28] In addition, in a retrospective observational study, ICU telemedicine services were deployed in Dehradun, India, as part of an attempt to improve cardiac critical care capabilities and specifically, the acute management of

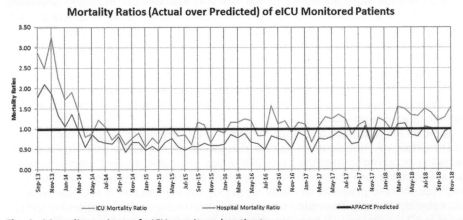

Fig. 1. Mortality rations of eICU monitored patients.

patients presenting with acute coronary syndrome. The implementation of an around-the-clock centralized tele-ICU program resulted in significant improvement in 30-day mortality rates (16.4% to 4.8%) along with improved time from door to needle/thrombolytic therapy for patients with ST-elevation myocardial infarctions.[29]

The US military has explored the utilization of ICU telemedicine capabilities as part of its deployments. This has been particularly explored for special forces operators who are often functioning in environments where their medics on the ground represent the most advanced medical provider available, and evacuation of critically ill patients to a more robust care environment may not be possible for a variety of reasons.[30] The Virtual Critical Care (VC3) Consult Service allows for on-demand virtual consultation with experienced critical care physicians. The service is accessed via a single phone line directly to an intensivist, and an email distribution list is used to pass information, including images, flowsheet data, and video clips.[30] Although not as efficient as some of the current civilian technology, particularly from a video or data transfer perspective, cellular telephone-based communication with e-mail supplementation is preferred because of its low bandwidth, minimal equipment requirements, and near-universal familiarity (particularly the act of speaking into a phone).[30] This system was made operational in 2015 with predominant usage with Special Operations Command Africa and Special Operations Command Central. Cases addressed via this system have included penetrating abdominal trauma and complex wound closure. Reported outcomes have been good, and operators have expressed satisfaction with the system.[30,31]

The conflict in Syria has also recently served as an environment for the implementation of an ICU telemedicine system. Because of ongoing fighting, the Syrian Republic's modern medical facilities have been destroyed, and thousands of the country's physicians have been killed or fled the region as refugees.[32] Intact ICUs have been maintained at low capacity because of a lack of staffing also.[32,33] Moughrabieh and Weinert described the implementation of a tele-ICU program that was started in 2012 to help manage the ICU care of patients throughout different parts of the country.[33] It currently has expanded to a network of approximately 20 intensivists providing clinical support 24 hours a day, 365 days a year. This construct has several unique elements to it, particularly when compared with tele-ICU models in the United States. Implementation is rapid (2 months). Care is offered in areas without formal bureaucratic structure, minimizing accreditation and credentialing issues.[33,34] The total operating costs for this construct were noted to be much lower than traditional tele-ICU models due to clinicians donating their time and the use of a virtual network along with commercially available communication applications like WhatsApp.[33,34]

OPPORTUNITIES FOR INTENSIVE CARE UNIT TELEMEDICINE INNOVATION
A Role for the Advanced Practice Provider

ICU telemedicine is now established as a viable solution for delivering ICU care in resource-limited environments and in the face of intensivist staffing shortfalls. There are other opportunities that could be explored to enhance delivery and effectiveness further. One such area is the integration of APPs in the ICU telemedicine environment, serving a clinical role behind the camera.

APPs have been integrated into ICUs as alternative physician trainees (permanent house staff) to offer direct yet supervised management of critically ill patients.[35] This integration improves adherence to coordination of care while not harming specific subgroups of patients.[36,37] It is cost-effective while maintaining or even improving the length of stay and mortality.[35,38,39] Coupling APPs with an ICU telemedicine program has also been associated with significant cost savings.[40]

A centralized continuous care model is a common ICU telemedicine delivery structure.[41,42] This is realized with a remote physical site (the hub) colocating physicians, nurses, and clerical staff who are connected (the spokes) to distant ICUs[41] Within this model, which tends to operate in 24/7/365 fashion, nurses are responsible for providing intense monitoring of between 35 and 45 patients, enabling a collaborating physician to serve up to 250 geographically dispersed patients.[42] As a program grows to include patients with greater and lesser needs, a valuable role for an experienced, critical care advanced practice provider can evolve. Low-acuity issues and routine activities (eg, correcting common electrolyte abnormalities) that otherwise absorb a physician's time could be handled quickly and efficiently by the APP, similar to the division of labor now common in a brick-and-mortar ICU construct. This would be particularly beneficial for ICUs that do not have surrogate providers immediately available at the bedside. Experienced APPs can take on progressive responsibilities, especially in times that an attending tele-intensivist is addressing crises, which are common when covering multiple ICUs. Lags in plans of care (both their creation and approval) would diminish – and coordination with bedside teams will likely accelerate –with the addition of an APP in this role and thus further enhance the capabilities and effectiveness of the centralized continuous care model.

Advanced Machine Learning and Alerting

ICU telemedicine delivers a significant benefit via real-time assessment of physiology and sophisticated trend-based and Boolean alerts.[7] Although bedside teams are structured to be aware of and to respond to bedside alarms, it is not uncommon for alarms to be missed, often because of ongoing alarm fatigue. The consequences of missed alerts are important; ICUs with reported response times to physiologic alerts of less than 3 minutes have significantly shorter ICU length of stays compared with those reporting longer response times.[43] ICU telemedicine support has an effect here as well, as without it, bedside nursing response to 90% of alarms for physiologic instability within 3 minutes of their onset occurs in only 45% of ICUs. Once implemented, ICU telemedicine support that incorporates these more advanced alerting tools has enabled 71% of ICUs to reach the 3 minutes or fewer goal.[44] The authors hasten to add that remote evaluation and adjudication of alerts cannot and will not replace essential bedside responses and responders to immediate life threats such as ventricular tachycardia alarms.

Clinical decision support tools are increasingly being utilized to help forecast a variety of conditions.[45,46] Many use static measurements harvested from the electronic medical record. Dynamic data, such as blood pressure and heart rate collected in real time, can augment predictive power.[47] Recent evidence has demonstrated that a prediction model derived from a combination of EMR data and high-frequency physiologic data (blood pressure and heart rate) can be utilized to predict the onset of sepsis up to 4 hours in advance of its presentation.[45]

These aspects of machine learning, combined with the architectures of ICU telemedicine systems built for robust and consistent response to physiologic alerts, offer a unique opportunity to further enhance and streamline critical care. Running a clinical decision support tool within the background of an ICU telemedicine system that is already equipped to gather real-time physiologic data as well as recognize and prompt the adherence (or lack thereof) to best practices offers enormous potential.[21,48] In the case of sepsis, earlier identification about its pending development can be detected by the telemedicine ICU team and its framework of clinical decision support tools and then relayed to the bedside team prompting further evaluation and early, appropriate management such as volume resuscitation, antibiotic administration, and prompt source control. The authors hasten to add that all predictive tools, including advanced machine learning tools, depend on the reliable flow of high-quality data. Data interruption, confusion, and contamination erode automated analyses, and the authors strongly argue for the use of experienced alert adjudicators (the tele-critical care staff) as essential components in such decision support models.

Medical Education

Concern has been raised that the presence of ICU telemedicine and imagined micro-management might infringe upon the autonomy with which house-staff operate while within supervised academic environments.[8] This has not been borne out in the literature, and surveys of house-staff have indicated a positive experience with the technology and the education it has provided.[49,50] As attending intensivist staffing patterns remained strained and ACGME duty hours restrictions reduce trainee presence, critical care bedside education can be necessary at off hours. ICU telemedicine offers an extraordinary opportunity to advance the education of not only house-staff but also APP trainees. Utilizing the variety of real-time physiologic data and support systems that it has at hand, the ICU telemedicine intensivist can offer real-time feedback to resident and fellow trainees about a posited intervention while also reinforcing the importance of the implementation of best practices via real-time updates about missed opportunities.[8] Additional skill sets like ultrasound imaging attainment and interpretation can be delivered also.[51]

Bringing trainees into the ICU telemedicine hub and giving them time behind the camera represents another opportunity for innovative medical education. Exposure to the technology and its associated clinical decision support systems offers several opportunities for stimulating further exploration, including research questions and quality improvement projects. At the same time, it offers an opportunity for one-on-one education and discussion directly with an intensivist attending, which can often be difficult to attain within a busy yet dispersed brick and mortar ICU. Insight into operations, plans of care, and patient populations in ICUs in which regular on-the-ground rotations are not available can be beneficial and informative, as can providing care into more remote/community-based ICUs. Large numbers of patients enable assignment of disease-based cohorts to trainees. For example, it is simple to assign 24 patients with sepsis, or a similar number with atrial fibrillation, or a similar number with acute respiratory disease syndrome (ARDS), to a trainee on a given shift. At the authors' institution, elective rotations in the eICU with pulmonary/critical care fellows, anesthesia fellows, and surgical critical care fellows have been well received by faculty and trainees, and discussions are underway to formalize a standing rotation.

Turning Night into Day

Burnout syndromes are common in health care as a whole, and in critical care in particular.[52] Stressful situations, long hours, and night shift work all contribute to burnout. Sustained sleep deprivation can have enormous health consequences.[53] ICU telemedicine, often tasked with providing critical care coverage during the night hours, has the potential to relieve these stresses at the bedside and paradoxically be heavily affected. Indeed, few staff—whether assigned to the bedside or to the tele-health center—are excited about night shift work.

Because telecare is by definition "at a distance," it is up to the operators to determine just how distant the hub and staff should be located. Emory's eICU center has located part of its operations on the other side of the world, where the Georgia night-time corresponds to antipodal daytime. The authors recently completed a 6-month, proof-of-principle study with Macquarie University, where 4 critical care physicians and 3 critical care nurses serially rotated to Sydney, Australia. They delivered critical care during the day back to the Emory Healthcare System in Atlanta, where it was nighttime (**Fig. 2**). The program was well received, with reported improved levels of concentration, efficiency, and job satisfaction. More recently, the authors launched a second phase hosted by Royal Perth Hospital in Perth, Western Australia, which is a full 12- to 13-hour time difference (seasonal variation) from Atlanta, favoring optimal wake-work-sleep patterns.[54]

This element of globalization seeks to leverage the technology of ICU telemedicine and offers the continued provision of efficient and effective care while simultaneously combating direct hindrances to job satisfaction and the development of burnout. Given the ongoing worldwide spread of ICU telemedicine, it is possible that this endeavor represents the beginnings of a global critical care network providing collaborative coverage and serving as a springboard for future investigations.[8,25,26,33]

LIMITATIONS

ICU telemedicine has several limitations to its implementation. These are practically grouped into financial, organizational and behavioral, and technical issues, although there are overlaps among the groupings.

Financial Element

For most ICU telemedicine systems, a significant amount of capital is required for initiation, and this is often cited as a major barrier to its use.[55] Recent analyses have estimated the cost to initiate an ICU telemedicine program for 1 year to be between $50,000 and $123,000 (in 2011 US dollars) per each monitored ICU bed and with total operating costs extending up to $3 million annually.[56–58] The financial return on investment associated with ICU telemedicine has not been well defined in the literature.[59,60] Recent work by Lilly and colleagues, however, found that implementation of ICU

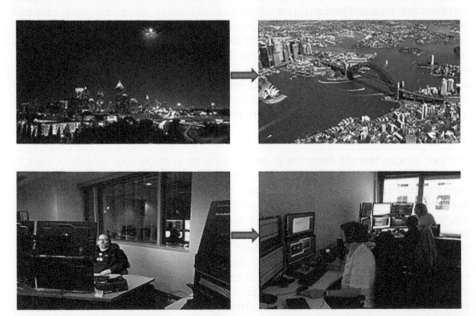

Fig. 2. Turning night into day.

telemedicine led to financial benefits that exceeded program capital and operating costs through increased case volume, higher case revenue relative to direct costs, and shorter length of stay.[59,60]

Another financial component that serves as a significant barrier is the reimbursement of services provided. In most cases, reimbursement is limited. In rare cases, reimbursement is provided at the standard rate of brick and mortar ICU care, despite the increased cost associated with the delivery of ICU telemedicine.[40] Category 3 (data collection) codes for ICU telemedicine services exist, but these costs are not currently reimbursed by the Centers for Medicare and Medicaid Services (CMS). At the same time, Medicare beneficiaries are eligible for telehealth services only if they are received at a site located in a rural Health Professional Shortage Area or in a county outside of a Metropolitan Statistical Area.[8]

Organizational and Behavioral Element

The acceptance of ICU telemedicine into an existing medical system relies on a shift of attitudes and the establishment of trust among all care providers. It is not uncommon for clinical providers at the bedside to feel threatened and scrutinized by telemedicine providers.[61] At the same time, the definitive role telemedicine providers are to play in a patient's care can be unclear at various points, and this can lead to disengagement. These difficulties can be particularly pointed in situations where the telemedicine team is providing care and support to a location very distant to its own. Several frequently cited elements that also contribute to this fractured construct include misunderstanding and faulty assumptions regarding onsite resources, equipment, and medication availability; unrealistic expectations about local staff education and abilities; lack of trust; and physician conflicts.[62]

It is not surprising then that robust communication between telemedicine providers and local clinicians can help address and eliminate these issues. Providing familiarity with both parties' workflows can allow a degree of trust and familiarity to develop.[63] At the same time, it needs to be recognized that many of the interactions that permeate ICU telemedicine need to be centered upon the simple tenets that serve as a hallmark for good customer service, notably respect, understanding, listening, responding, and serving. Being able to hold to these principles while concurrently discussing the management of a critically ill patient and navigating advanced technology is a skill set that not every provider will have, nor can they necessarily be taught to produce it repeatedly. It is key, then, to make sure that staff members are carefully vetted and chosen then adequately trained and educated prior to their deployment in an attempt to address this issue.

Technical Element

Not surprisingly, there is a significant technical limitation to ICU telemedicine also. In general, a substantial amount of manpower must be deployed to get an ICU telemedicine system installed, and more often than not, a large amount of sophisticated hardware must be fitted and set up.[61] Once installed, there are numerous upgrades and updates to software, and ensuring sustained interoperability between these elements and the electronic medical record system is important, time-consuming, and an often cited reason for choosing not to participate with ICU telemedicine.[57]

Maintenance and upkeep of specialized in-room equipment can require separate staffing and skill sets. Such skills must be gained on-site. Ensuring operability across multiple hospitals with appropriate data transfer is complex despite efforts to increase interoperability.[41] With increasing variability in product choices, it is necessary to have a robust understanding of both current and future needs, particularly in light of emerging technologies. This, again, requires advanced expertise and skill set different from that used by providers who use telemedicine systems on a daily basis to help deliver care.[41]

The globalization of critical care, particularly in ultra-long distance construct such as Emory's Night Into Day program, has created new challenges. Contemporary tele-critical care software and hardware use communication protocols within client-server architectures to transmit large quantities of data with each mouse click. So long as the clients are located near servers (ie, within a few hundred miles), the latencies associated with transmission and verification of the accuracy of each data packet prior to transmission of the next packet are imperceptible to clinicians. Once those distances extend to thousands of miles, however, those additional milliseconds add up to perceptible slowness. New software architectures will likely need to take advantage of cloud computing and virtual machines in order to fully globalize such remote care.

SUMMARY

ICU telemedicine represents a well-validated tool to help combat much of the demand that has been placed upon the field of critical care in recent years. Its capabilities to help alleviate heterogeneous intensivist staffing patterns in both the developed and developing world have served as a springboard for further innovations. There appears to be a growing role for APPs in ICU telemedicine along with a role for educating trainees both at the bedside and behind the computer screen. The integration of machine learning into daily ICU telemedicine practice offers new opportunities for the timely evaluation and management of complex conditions like sepsis. The computational infrastructure of ICU telemedicine promises robust globalization of critical care services.

REFERENCES

1. Buchman TG, Coopersmith CM, Meissen HW, et al. Innovative interdisciplinary strategies to address the intensivist shortage. Crit Care Med 2017; 45:298–304.
2. Angus DC, Kelley MA, Schmitz RJ, et al, Committee on Manpower for Pulmonary and Critical Care Societies (COMPACCS). Caring for the critically ill patient. Current and projected workforce requirements for care of the critically ill and patients with pulmonary disease: can we meet the requirements of an aging population? JAMA 2000;284:2762–70.
3. Ewart GW, Marcus L, Gaba MM, et al. The critical care medicine crisis: a call for federal action: a white paper from the critical care professional societies. Chest 2004;125:1518–21.
4. Health resources and services administration report to Congress: the critical care workforce: a study of the supply and demand for critical care physicians. 2006. Available at: http://bhpr.hrsa.gov/healthworkforce/reports/studycriticalcarephys.pdf. Accessed November 22, 2018.
5. Halpern NA, Goldman DA, Tan KS, et al. Trends in critical care beds and use among population groups and Medicare and Medicaid beneficiaries in the United States: 2000–2010. Crit Care Med 2016;44:1490–9.
6. Kahn JM. ICU telemedicine: from theory to practice. Crit Care Med 2014;42: 2457–8.
7. Fuhrman SA, Lilly CM. ICU telemedicine solutions. Clin Chest Med 2015;36(3): 401–7.

8. Lilly CM, Zubrow MT, Kempner KM, et al. Society of critical care medicine tele-ICU Committee. Critical care telemedicine: evolution and state of the art. Crit Care Med 2014;42(11):2429–36.

9. Reynolds HN, Bander JJ. Options for tele-intensive care unit design: centralized versus decentralized and other considerations: it is not just a "another black sedan." Crit Care Clin 2015;31(2):335–50.

10. Phillips eICU program. Available at: https://www.usa.philips.com/healthcare/product/HC865325ICU/eicu-program-telehealth-for-the-intensive-care-unit. Accessed January 8, 2019.

11. InTouch Health. Available at: https://intouchhealth.com/virtual-care-platform/intouch-os/. Accessed January 8, 2019.

12. PeraHealth. Available at: https://www.perahealth.com/. Accessed January 8, 2019.

13. BedMasterEx. Available at: https://www.bedmaster.net/en/products/bedmasterex. Accessed January 8, 2019.

14. Cox P, Willis K, Coustasse A. (2014, March). The American epidemic: The U.S. nursing shortage and turnover problem. Paper presented at BHAA 2014, Chicago, IL, March 26, 2014.

15. American Association of Colleges of Nursing. Nursing faculty shortage Fact Sheet 2017. 2018. Available at: https://www.aacnnursing.org/News-Information/Fact-Sheets/Nursing-Faculty-Shortage. Accessed January 2, 2019.

16. Kelley MA, Angus D, Chalfin DB, et al. The critical care crisis in the United States: a report from the profession. Chest 2004;125:1514–7.

17. Rosenfeld BA, Dorman T, Breslow MJ, et al. Intensive care unit telemedicine: alternate paradigm for providing continuous intensivist care. Crit Care Med 2000;28:3925–31.

18. American Heart Association. Fast facts on US hospitals 2018. Available at: https://www.aha.org/statistics/fast-facts-us-hospitals. Accessed November 1, 2018.

19. Zawada ET Jr, Herr P, Larson D, et al. Impact of an intensive care unit telemedicine program on a rural health care system. Postgrad Med 2009;121(3):160–70.

20. Zawada ET Jr, Kapaska D, Herr P, et al. Prognostic outcomes after the initiation of an electronic telemedicine intensive care unit (EICU) in a rural health system. S D Med 2006;59(9):391–3.

21. Lilly CM, Cody S, Zhao H, et al. Hospital mortality, length of stay, and preventable complications among critically ill patients before and after tele-ICU reengineering of critical care processes. JAMA 2011;305(21):2175–83.

22. Fusaro MV, Becker C, Scurlock C. Evaluating tele-ICU implementation based on observed and predicted ICU mortality: a systematic review and meta-analysis. Crit Care Med 2019;47(4):501–7.

23. Sturman C. Phillips launches a tele-intensive care eICU programme in Japan. 2018. Available at: https://www.healthcareglobal.com/public-health/philips-launches-tele-intensive-care-eicu-programme-japan. Accessed November 20, 2018.

24. Philips delivers the Middle East's first TeleICU program in collaboration with UAE Ministry of Health. Available at: https://www.albawaba.com/business/pr/philips-delivers-middle-east%E2%80%99s-first-teleicu-program-collaboration-uae-ministry-health-8. Accessed November 20, 2018.

25. GE Healthcare, Fortis pioneer Asia's first eICU. 2012. Available at: https://www.biospectrumasia.com/news/27/3769/ge-healthcare-fortis-pioneer-asias-first-eicu.html. Accessed November 22, 2018.

26. Fortis healthcare EICU. 2018. Available at: https://www.fortishealthcare.com/eicu. Accessed November, 22, 2018.

27. Gupta S, Kaushal A, Dewan S, et al. Can an electronic ICU support timely renal replacement therapy in resource-limited areas of the developing world. Crit Care 2015;19(Suppl 1):P504.

28. Kaushal A, Gupta S, Dewan S, et al. India's first tele-ICU: critinext. Crit Care Med 2013;41(12):A147.

29. Gupta S, Dewan S, Kaushal A, et al. eICU reduces mortality in STEMI patients in resource-limited areas. Glob Heart 2014;9:425–7.

30. Powell D, McLeroy RD, Riesberg J, et al. Telemedicine to reduce medical risk in austere medical environments: the virtual critical care consultation (VC3) service. J Spec Oper Med 2016;16(4):102–9.

31. DellaVolpe J, Lantry J, Powell D, et al. The role of virtual critical care consultation in supporting military combat operations. Crit Care Med 2016;44(12):468.

32. Ahsan S. In Syria, doctors beware. New York Times 2013. Available at: http://www.nytimes.com/2013/10/04/opinion/in-syria-doctors-beware.html. Accessed November 22, 2018.

33. Moughrabieh A, Weinert C. Rapid deployment of international tele–intensive care unit services in War-Torn Syria. Ann Am Thorac Soc 2016;13(2):165–72.

34. Moughrabieh M, Weinert C, Zaza T. Rapid deployment of international tele-ICU services during conflict in Syria. Am J Respir Crit Care Med 2014;189:A3630.

35. Gershengorn HB, Johnson MP, Factor P. The use of nonphysician providers in adult intensive care units. Am J Respir Crit Care Med 2012;185(6):600–5.

36. Hoffman LA, Tasota FJ, Scharfenberg C, et al. Management of patients in the intensive care unit: comparison via work sampling analysis of an acute care nurse practitioner and physicians in training. Am J Crit Care 2003;12:436–43.

37. Hoffman LA, Miller TH, Zullo TG, et al. Comparison of 2 models for managing tracheotomized patients in a subacute medical intensive care unit. Respir Care 2006;51:1230–6.

38. Fry M. Literature review of the impact of nurse practitioners in critical care services. Nurs Crit Care 2011;16(2):58–66.

39. Kleinpell RM, Ely W, Grabenkort R. Nurse practitioners and physician assistants in the intensive care unit: an evidence-based review. Crit Care Med 2008;36(10):2888–97.

40. Trombley MJ, Hassol A, Lloyd JT, et al. The impact of enhanced critical care training and 24/7 (Tele-ICU) support on medicare spending and postdischarge utilization patterns. Health Serv Res 2018;53:2099–117.

41. Reynolds HN, Rogove H, Joseph Bander J, et al. A working lexicon for the tele-intensive care unit: we need to define tele-intensive care unit to grow and understand it. Telemed J E Health 2011;17(10):773–83.

42. Davis TM, Barden C, Dean S, et al. American telemedicine association guidelines for TeleICU operations. Telemed J E Health 2016;22(12):971–80.

43. Lilly CM, McLaughlin JM, Zhao H, et al. A multicenter study of ICU telemedicine reengineering of adult critical care. Chest 2014;145:500–7.

44. Lilly CM, Fisher KA, Ries M, et al. A national ICU telemedicine survey: validation and results. Chest 2012;142:40–7.

45. Nemati S, Holder A, Razmi F, et al. An interpretable machine learning model for accurate prediction of sepsis in the ICU. Crit Care Med 2018;46(4):547–53.

46. Koyner JL, Carey KA, Edelson DP, et al. The development of a machine learning inpatient acute kidney injury prediction model. Crit Care Med 2018;46(7):1070–7.

47. Mayaud L, Lai PS, Clifford GD, et al. Dynamic data during hypotensive episode improves mortality predictions among patients with sepsis and hypotension. Crit Care Med 2013;41:954–62.
48. Kahn JM, Gunn SR, Lorenz HL, et al. Impact of nurse-led remote screening and prompting for evidence-based practices in the ICU. Crit Care Med 2014;42: 896–904.
49. Coletti C, Elliott DJ, Zubrow MT. Resident perceptions of a teleintensive care unit implementation. Telemed J E Health 2010;16:894–7.
50. Mora A, Faiz SA, Kelly T, et al. Resident perception of the educational and patient care value from remote telemonitoring in a medical intensive care unit. Chest 2007;132:443A.
51. Levine AR, McCurdy MT, Zubrow MT, et al. Tele-intensivists can instruct non-physicians to acquire high-quality ultrasound images. J Crit Care 2015;30(5): 871–5.
52. Moss M, Good VS, Gozal D, et al. An official critical care societies collaborative statement: burnout syndrome in critical care healthcare professionals a call for action. Crit Care Med 2016;44(7):1414–21.
53. Haus EL, Smolensky MH. Shift work and cancer risk: potential mechanistic roles of circadian disruption, light at night, and sleep deprivation. Sleep Med Rev 2013; 17:273–84.
54. Emory cares for ICU patients remotely, turning 'night into day' from Australia. Available at: http://news.emory.edu/stories/2018/05/buchman-hiddleson_eicu_perth_australia//. Accessed November 1, 2018.
55. Berenson RA, Grossman JM, November EA. Does telemonitoring of patients–the eICU–improve intensive care? Health Aff 2009;28:w937–47.
56. Kumar G, Falk DM, Bonello RS, et al. The costs of critical care telemedicine programs: a systematic review and analysis. Chest 2013;143:19–29.
57. Lilly CM, Motzkus C, Rincon T, et al, UMass Memorial Critical Care Operations Group. ICU telemedicine program financial outcomes. Chest 2017;151:286–97.
58. Coustasse A, Deslich S, Bailey D, et al. A business case for tele-intensive care units. Perm J 2014;18:76–84.
59. Lilly CM, Motzkus CA. ICU telemedicine: financial analyses of a complex intervention. Crit Care Med 2017;45:1558–61.
60. Vranas KC, Slatore CG, Kerlin MP. Telemedicine coverage of intensive care units: a narrative review. Ann Am Thorac Soc 2018;15(11):1256–64.
61. Avdalovic MV, Marcin JP. When will telemedicine appear in the ICU? J Intensive Care Med 2018;34(4):271–6.
62. Wilkes MS, Marcin JP, Ritter LA, et al. Organizational and teamwork factors of tele-intensive care units. Am J Crit Care 2016;25(5):431–9.
63. Moeckli J, Cram P, Cunningham C, et al. Staff acceptance of a telemedicine intensive care unit program: a qualitative study. J Crit Care 2013;28(6):890–901.

Satisfaction in Intensive Care Unit Telemedicine Programs

Annie B. Johnson, MSN, CNP*

KEYWORDS

- ICU telemedicine program • Satisfaction • Tele-ICU • eICU

KEY POINTS

- Measuring satisfaction in an ICU telemedicine program is multifaceted, therefore making it more difficult to measure than may first be presumed.
- There is not yet a tool that has been developed or universally used to assess satisfaction within ICU telemedicine programs.
- Effective communication is commonly highlighted as a significant contributor to satisfaction in ICU telemedicine programs.

INTRODUCTION

Telemedicine has been used for many years to enhance the bedside care of critically ill patients. Naturally the implementation of such a service, whether on the providing or receiving end, generates inquiries about outcomes. Among the outcomes that are measured, perhaps one of the most important yet difficult to capture is the measurement of satisfaction. This article describes ways in which organizations can evaluate patient and provider satisfaction, factors that may affect satisfaction, and standards to consider when measuring patient and provider satisfaction in an intensive care unit (ICU) telemedicine (tele-ICU) program.

TOOLS FOR EVALUATING PATIENT AND PROVIDER SATISFACTION IN AN INTENSIVE CARE UNIT TELEMEDICINE PROGRAM

Measuring satisfaction in a tele-ICU program is multifaceted, therefore making it more difficult to measure than may first be presumed. One must not only consider the

Disclosure Statement: The author has no relationship with a commercial company that has a direct financial interest in subject matter or materials discussed in this article or with a company making a competing product.
Department of Pulmonary and Critical Care Medicine, Mayo Clinic, Rochester, MN, USA
* 200 1st Street SW, Rochester, MN 55902.
E-mail address: walker.andrea@mayo.edu

satisfaction of the patient, family, nurse, and physician on the receiving end of the care but also the satisfaction of the tele-ICU nurse and physician. What creates desirable levels of satisfaction on one end may not necessarily translate into the same levels of satisfaction on the other.

There is not yet a validated tool that has been specifically developed to measure satisfaction within a tele-ICU program. Many of the studies that have been done to capture this measurement have used self-created surveys administered to staff.[1–3] In addition to surveys, interviews conducted via phone calls as well as site visits were also reported as a means of gathering information related to staff perception of the tele-ICU.[1] An advantage of these tools is that they can be expressly tailored to the specific tele-ICU services that are being studied, thus uncovering more nuanced details that a universal approach may not.

There have been studies that used validated tools, adapting them to study tele-ICU satisfaction more accurately. Kleinpell and colleagues[4] used the eICU Acceptance Survey adapting it to further evaluate nursing perception on the barriers and benefits that telemedicine creates in regard to nursing care. A team from Johns Hopkins Hospital explored the perceptions of the bedside nurse in regard to a tele-ICU service by using a validated survey employed in a prior study to understand bedside provider perceptions.[5] Other investigators have chosen to use tools such as the Safety Climate Scale (SCS) and Teamwork Climate Scale (TCS) because of their correlation with patient outcomes, although even these scales had been heavily amended to more accurately represent perceptions of tele-ICU programs (Appendix 1).[6]

Of the studies reviewed for this article, only one specifically detailed the satisfaction of the patient and family in regard to the tele-ICU survey.[7] This study used the Schmidt Perception of Nursing Care Survey (SPNCS), a validated survey that assesses the overall hospital experience of the patient and family based on the perception of the nursing care provided. With permission, the authors of this study amended the survey to assess the staff as a whole by changing the words "nursing" to "staff," and also by adding 3 additional questions that specifically explored patient and family perceptions of the tele-ICU.[7]

Overall, satisfaction with regard to tele-ICU programs remains a difficult outcome to capture. Studies using customized surveys are informative and help to identify common themes that may emerge. However, it will continue to be challenging to hold tele-ICU programs to a set standard regarding satisfaction without the development of a widely used, reliable, and validated survey.

FACTORS THAT AFFECT SATISFACTION

Measuring satisfaction in a tele-ICU environment is unique in that there are 2 groups of staff to consider during the comprehensive assessment of satisfaction. One needs to be focused on both the staff providing the tele-ICU service and the staff who interface with the service, also known as the spoke site. Of course, understanding factors that affect satisfaction from all sides will ultimately be reflected in the measured satisfaction of the patients and families who interact with the tele-ICU program. There now follows a discussion of the main themes identified in the reviewed studies regarding factors that contribute to satisfaction by the aforementioned stakeholders (**Fig. 1**).

Communication

No matter which side of the tele-ICU program one is on, communication is commonly highlighted as a contributor to satisfaction. A study by Hoonakker and colleagues[8] looked at the trust and satisfaction levels that nurses who worked in the telemedicine

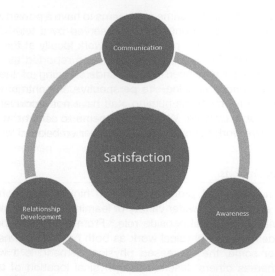

Fig. 1. The 3 key aspects of satisfaction as it relates to intensive care unit telemedicine programs.

ICU had with the bedside nurses at the spoke site, whereby 3 themes became very clear: openness, accuracy, and timeliness of communication. The more open, accurate, and timely the communication back from the bedside registered nurse at the spoke site, the higher the trust and satisfaction the telemedicine registered nurse had with the bedside nurse. This communication loop is important to be maintained also in the other direction. Nurses at the spoke site find it very important that changes in the plan of care or updates on their patients be communicated directly with them as well as with the physician.[9] Failure to do so risks damaging the professional relationship that is vital to the success of the tele-ICU program.

Communication among hospital administration and the staff of both the tele-ICU program and the spoke sites is also important in regard to satisfaction, both during the development phase of these programs and in an ongoing manner. Both physicians and nurses relay that job satisfaction within this role depends heavily on understanding the role and expectations through proper training, sharing in the perceived need of the service, and organization with standards and protocols put in place from an operational standpoint.[10] Communication is the key to all items already mentioned.

Relationships

The relationship, closely linked to communication, is another factor contributing to satisfaction within tele-ICU programs. The relationship between the nursing staff and telemedicine physician is quoted as being very important for both the telemedicine service and the spoke sites. Two separate studies indicated that it was important for the bedside nurses to know the telemedicine physician they were working with.[8,9] It has also been described that telemedicine nurses feel they are able to develop closer professional relationships with the physicians in the program than they are able to have in a more traditional hierarchal setting, contributing to higher levels of satisfaction.[8,9]

The importance of relationships on satisfaction is likewise echoed by reports that telemedicine nurses have higher levels of satisfaction with and trust in their spoke-site counterparts if they had or continue to work at the bedside of these sites.[3]

Physically working together on the same unit seems to have a powerful impact on relationship building. This has been anecdotally observed by a tele-ICU program that temporarily assigned telemedicine physicians to work locally at the interfacing sites during staffing shortages. The result of this has been reported as high satisfaction by the physicians and an enhanced mutual understanding of the workflow both from the telemedicine and interfacing-site perspective. In contrast to this, observational site visits by the telemedicine nursing staff have not produced the same level of enhanced relationship building. What really seems to affect the most change is engaging in productive work hours as a staff member embedded within the sites.

Professional Considerations

Nurses working in a tele-ICU program describe high satisfaction with their role because they are exposed to a wider variety of learning opportunities than they may otherwise have with a traditional bedside role.[8] From a workflow perspective, telemedicine nurses describe the physical work as both positive and negative in regard to satisfaction. For some, the decreased physical demand is a welcome change and a satisfier whereas others describe the physical location of the tele-ICU (eg, lack of windows and natural light, prolonged sitting) as a negative.[8] Other workflow issues that have been identified include telemedicine nurses missing the hands-on experiences with patients and families and high workloads with upward of 40 patients to be accountable for.[8]

Similar to the nursing staff, telemedicine physicians found this work to be mentally challenging but less physically so. They reported this work to be beneficial in that it provides access to critical care in regional areas where it is typically difficult to provide appropriate care.[11] The physicians also saw this as an additional opportunity to extend their critical care careers and did not report any adverse effects on their current bedside practice or patient care.[11]

The staff of the spoke sites has varying role-dependent perspectives on the impact of the workflow. Thus, satisfaction is also variable. Physicians of the spoke sites found that the tele-ICU program lessened the burden of caring for patients, whereas the bedside nurses at these sites tended to have a different perception.[1] The nurses were more affected by more substantial amounts of orders to implement than by whether the local provider was caring for the patient. Therefore, the burden of work was not entirely as lessened for the nursing staff as the physicians had indicated.[1] Spoke-site nurses also reported the interruption in workflow by the telemedicine service and the risk of feeling "spied upon" if not made aware of the on-camera presence, thus affecting satisfaction with the service, all of which could arguably be mitigated through more effective communication.[8]

Another theme that has emerged in the literature in regard to satisfaction with tele-ICU programs is related to the amount of interaction that the spoke sites had with the program. Hospitals that had interacted with a tele-ICU program for a longer duration and interacted with the service more frequently were more satisfied with the service.[1] Related to this is the finding that the more hours the tele-ICU nurses worked each week, the higher was their reported satisfaction.[3] However, even if the interactions between spoke sites with the tele-ICU program were not significant from a time or frequency perspective, spoke-site staff remained satisfied with the service when there was a critically ill patient present who could not be transferred to a higher level of care.[1] This reality seems to reinforce that the perception of usefulness and the ability to create a real impact on medical practice is a strong satisfier for those involved with tele-ICU programs.[1,10]

Patient and Family

In reviewing the literature on satisfaction as it relates to tele-ICU programs, it is quickly apparent that little has been done to specifically study the satisfaction of the patient and family with these programs. As previously described, Golembeski and colleagues[7] explored patient and family perceptions of a tele-ICU program, both before and after implementation. This study illustrates that the most significant factor influencing satisfaction of patients and family members was the awareness that the care team was on site as well as remote in the tele-ICU. This finding circles back to and connects with the influence of the other previously discussed factors of effective communication and building trusting relationships.

STANDARDS FOR MEASURING SATISFACTION IN AN INTENSIVE CARE UNIT TELEMEDICINE PROGRAM

Given that there is not yet a tool that has been developed or universally used to assess satisfaction within tele-ICU programs, it is no surprise that there are also no clearly defined standards through which tele-ICU programs can compare themselves regarding satisfaction. However, national organizations such as the American Association of Critical Care Nurses (AACN) have begun to address this.

In 2013, the AACN published practice guidelines titled "AACN Tele-ICU Nursing Practice Guidelines" with the goal of defining the tele-ICU nursing service and to guide programs as a whole using the essential aspects of telemedicine care as well as means by which to evaluate the individual practice (AACN, 2013). This mostly allowed the organizations developing tele-ICU programs to define the outcomes based on their own site-specific goals with a varying focus on performance evaluation. In many instances this may be appropriate given that tele-ICU programs exist for a variety of different reasons and provide unique needs to those they serve.

However, in regard to outcomes on satisfaction, there are standards to which traditional critical care practices are held that can inform these same outcomes for tele-ICU programs. In 2005, the AACN developed an initiative to create and sustain healthy work environments in response to reports that unhealthy work environments contributed to poor patient outcomes because of events such as medication errors and infection rates.[12] Of the 6 standards that were developed through this initiative, 3 were highlighted explicitly in regard to tele-ICU programs and the receiving sites: skilled communication, true collaboration, and effective decision making.[12] These 3 standards are aligned very closely with the previous discussion regarding factors that contribute to satisfaction in tele-ICU programs.

Influential organizations such as The Joint Commission and the National Quality Forum have established recommendations that an organization's climate of safety be measured annually through the use of tools such as the safety climate scale (SCS).[6] Other measurements of attributes such as teamwork, measured by the teamwork climate scale (TCS), have also been linked to benefits such as better patient outcomes and higher retention rates of nurses.[6] Again, one could extrapolate that high levels of safety and a strong sense of teamwork will translate to desirable levels of satisfaction.

The lack of defined standards with which to evaluate tele-ICU programs in regard to satisfaction does not necessarily mean that this cannot be adequately measured. Using guidelines and tools developed by organizations and commissions that establish standards and measure outcomes that are very closely aligned with satisfaction would be a very logical place for programs to start.

SUMMARY

For well over a decade, tele-ICU programs have been providing care to patients and families as well as an invaluable service to many receiving sites that are otherwise beyond the traditional reach of high-quality critical care. As technology advances and the population continues to age and grow, the scope of tele-ICU will only continue to expand. It will be important that during this growth, important outcomes regarding the unique services provided by tele-ICU services are accurately measured, not the least of which is nursing, provider, and patient and family satisfaction. More work is yet to be done to ensure that the voices of those most intimately affected by tele-ICU services are heard and that programs are evaluated and adapted in response to these outcomes.

REFERENCES

1. Ward MM, Ullrich F, Potter AJ, et al. Factors affecting staff perceptions of tele-ICU service in rural hospitals. Telemed J E Health 2015;21:459–66.
2. Otero AV, Lopez-Magallon AJ, Jaimes D, et al. International telemedicine in pediatric cardiac critical care: a multicenter experience. Telemed J E Health 2014;20: 619–25.
3. Hoonakker PLT, Pecanac KE, Brown RL, et al. Virtual collaboration, satisfaction, and trust between nurses in the tele-ICU and ICUs: results of a multilevel analysis. J Crit Care 2017;37:224–9.
4. Kleinpell R, Barden C, Rincon T, et al. Assessing the impact of telemedicine on nursing care in intensive care units. Am J Crit Care 2016;25:e14–20.
5. Romig MC, Latif A, Gill RS, et al. Perceived benefit of a telemedicine consultative service in a highly staffed intensive care unit. J Crit Care 2012;27:426.e9-16.
6. Chu-Weininger MY, Wueste L, Lucke JF, et al. The impact of a tele-ICU on provider attitudes about teamwork and safety climate. Qual Saf Health Care 2010; 19:e39.
7. Golembeski S, Willmitch B, Kim SS. Perceptions of the care experience in critical care units enhanced by a tele-ICU. AACN Adv Crit Care 2012;23:323–9.
8. Hoonakker PL, Carayon P, McGuire K, et al. Motivation and job satisfaction of Tele-ICU nurses. J Crit Care 2013;28:315.e13-21.
9. Mullen-Fortino M, DiMartino J, Entrikin L, et al. Bedside nurses' perceptions of intensive care unit telemedicine. Am J Crit Care 2012;21:24–31 [quiz: 32].
10. Moeckli J, Cram P, Cunningham C, et al. Staff acceptance of a telemedicine intensive care unit program: a qualitative study. J Crit Care 2013;28:890–901.
11. Zawada ET Jr, Herr P, Larson D, et al. Impact of an intensive care unit telemedicine program on a rural health care system. Postgrad Med 2009;121:160–70.
12. Goran SF, Mullen-Fortino M. Partnership for a healthy work environment: tele-ICU/ ICU collaborative. AACN Adv Crit Care 2012;23:289–301.

APPENDIX 1: TEAMWORK CLIMATE SCALE AND SAFETY CLIMATE SCALE ITEMS
Teamwork Climate
1. Nurse input is well received in this clinical area.
2. In this clinical area, it is difficult to speak up if I perceive a problem with patient care.
3. The physicians and nurses here work together as a well-coordinated team.
4. Disagreements in this clinical area are resolved appropriately.
5. It is easy for personnel here to ask questions when there is something they do not understand.
6. I have the support I need from other personnel to care for patients.

Safety Climate
1. I would feel safe being treated here as a patient.
2. I am encouraged by my colleagues to report any patient safety concerns I may have.
3. The culture in this clinical area makes it easy to learn from the errors of others.
4. I receive appropriate feedback about my performance.
5. Medical errors are handled appropriately here.
6. I know the proper channels to direct questions regarding patient safety in this clinical area.
7. In this clinical area, it is difficult to discuss errors.

Expansion of Telemedicine Services
Telepharmacy, Telestroke, Teledialysis, Tele–Emergency Medicine

Sandra L. Kane-Gill, PharmD, MSc, FCCM, FCCP[a],*,
Fred Rincon, MD, MSc, MBE, FCCP, FCCM[b]

KEYWORDS

- Critical care • Pharmaceutical care • Intensive care unit • Telemedicine
- Telepharmacy • Telestroke

KEY POINTS

- Telepharmacy offers an efficient expansion of services, in particular for hospitals that may not have the expertise of critical care–trained pharmacists.
- Telestroke provides efficacy in stroke recognition, image interpretation, increased intravenous administration of tissue plasminogen activator, and recognition of patients suitable for endovascular interventions.
- Tele-emergency services may be used to enhance patient care for circulatory injuries, respiratory distress, toxicologic events, and trauma.

INTRODUCTION

More than 50% of acute care hospitals use some form of telemedicine, and this rate is expected to grow by 20% to 50% each year.[1,2] In 2020, the cost of telehealth is expected to reach $34 billion.[3] The use of telemedicine is expanding into multiple subsets including tele–intensive care unit (tele-ICU) services. There are other subsets of telemedicine for acute care, such as pharmacy, stroke, and dialysis. The American Telemedicine Association (ATA) provides descriptions of the types of telemedicine, and of communication and models of care.[4,5] **Table 1**[4–8] provides a summary of various types of telemedicine. This article describes the subsets of telemedicine used for acute care.

Disclosure: S. Kane-Gill and F. Rincon have no financial disclosures.
[a] University of Pittsburgh, PUH/SHY Pharmacy Administration Building, 3507 Victoria Street, Mailcode PFG-01-01-01, Pittsburgh, PA 15213, USA; [b] Department of Neurosurgery, Thomas Jefferson University, 909 Walnut Street, 3rd Floor, Philadelphia, PA 19107, USA
* Corresponding author.
E-mail address: Kane-Gill@pitt.edu

Crit Care Clin 35 (2019) 519–533
https://doi.org/10.1016/j.ccc.2019.02.007
0749-0704/19/© 2019 Elsevier Inc. All rights reserved.

Table 1
Types of telemedicine and communication with examples

Type of Telemedicine	Definition	Type of Communication	Model of Care	Mode of Communication	Related Example
Store and forward	Forward and share medical data with a provider or patient at a different location	Asynchronous so that the patient and provider do not need to be communicating in real time	Responsive or scheduled	Secure e-mail platform	Monitoring glucose for a diabetic patient who stores data for a specified time period and then transmits information to the clinician Receiving medication orders for a patient in the hospital and forwarding the data to a remote pharmacist. The storing in this scenario is shorter than for an outpatient setting
Remote patient monitoring	Technology to record and transmit patient data automatically	Asynchronous so that the patient and provider do not need to be communicating in real time	Continuous monitoring with responsive or scheduled communication. Often clinician can transmit feedback and recommendations via the same mobile device on which the information was received	Mobile devices with bluetooth or radio frequency identification transmit data to a central control center for the clinician to review	Electrocardiogram monitoring or blood pressure monitoring The format adopted for electronic ICUs where data including medication information are continuously under surveillance

| Real-time telemedicine | Permitting 2-way, real-time, interactive communication between patients and clinicians who are geographically separated | Synchronous so that the patients and providers are communicating in real time | Responsive or scheduled | Telephonic or mobile device with video conferencing software | All types of clinical care, including telepharmacy, telestroke, and teledialysis |

Data from Refs.[4-8]

TELEPHARMACY

Tele-ICU services are viewed by clinicians as a way to improve evidence-based medicine compliance and support medication management that promotes the use of telepharmacy.[9] Telepharmacy is defined as the "provision of pharmacist care by registered pharmacies and pharmacists located within U.S. jurisdictions through the use of telecommunications or other technologies to patients or their agents at distances that are located within U.S. jurisdictions" according to the Model for State Pharmacy Act and Models Rules of the National Association of Boards of Pharmacy.[10] This definition is provided by an independent, international, and impartial association, but it is specific to services offered in the United States and has the potential for global application. Telepharmacy has been described as 4 types: (1) traditional full-service pharmacy, (2) remote consultation site, (3) hospital telepharmacy, and (4) automated dispensing machine controlled by a remote pharmacist.[11] Telepharmacy has primarily been studied in the outpatient setting, resulting in positive clinical outcomes.[12] The adoption of telepharmacy for inpatient care lags slightly behind that of telemedicine with a paucity of literature, especially for critically ill patients. Established telemedicine services in the ICU have added telepharmacy consultations.[13,14] The goal of telepharmacy services for critically ill patients includes (1) reaching patients that would not typically receive services, usually because of inadequate resources; (2) efficiently expanding services, as in the case of providing after-hours care; and (3) maintaining optimal patient care by having a pharmacist in the same remote location as the other members of the telemedicine health care team. For example, a health system extended services to smaller hospitals and provided after-hours care for 246 ICU beds at 13 hospitals by having pharmacists in the same off-site location as other members of the health care team.[15] Drivers for the implementation of critical care telepharmacy are similar to those for outpatient telepharmacy and remote clinical services provided for other reasons. Another objective of telepharmacy provided outside of the inpatient setting is dispensing medications; however, the pharmacists providing critical care services located in remote settings are not in a position to expeditiously dispense medications for immediate patient care.[15] Pharmacists providing critical care services are available to facilitate the medication dispensing by verifying medication orders if the technology is established to transmit the data.

Strnad and colleagues[16] provide a review of telepharmacy for ICU and non-ICU inpatient services and report the impact on patient outcomes for studies that used quasiexperimental designs. Overall, the investigators reported a positive impact on patient outcomes, nursing satisfaction, and disease management for 11 studies, including 3 ICU-specific evaluations. **Table 2**[13–15,17,18] provides an overview of telepharmacy services provided in the ICU for publications without restriction to study design with the goal of summarizing the services provided. Telepharmacy services combine a real-time process and store-and-forward technology. The type of communication is synchronous and asynchronous, typically dependent on the urgency of the communication. Responsive telephonic communication is used more frequently than video conferencing, although a scheduled video conferencing approach has been used as part of routine tele-ICU patient care rounds.[14]

Telepharmacy offers the advantage of efficiently expanding services, in particular to smaller hospitals that may not have the expertise of critical care–trained pharmacists for after-hours care. Pharmacists as part of an interdisciplinary team in the ICU have been shown to optimize patient outcomes and reduce adverse drug events.[19–21] Telepharmacy therefore offers a remote interdisciplinary team that includes the pharmacist where tele-ICU is provided.[14] The possible risks associated with telepharmacy are the

Table 2
Summary of publications describing telepharmacy services offered in the intensive care unit

Reference	Type of Telepharmacy	Type of Communication	Model of Care	Mode of Communication	Pharmacy Service Provided
Keeys et al,[17] 2002	Real-time telemedicine for high-priority communication Store and forward since medication orders were transmitted to the telepharmacist via facsimile	Asynchronous and synchronous	Responsive to request for consultation by physician or nurse about medications Responsive to problems identified during medication order review	Telephone or facsimile	Review of medication orders by a pharmacist, drug information, and clinical pharmacy consultations Service provided to the institution but prioritized new admissions and orders for patients transferred in and out of the ICU
Meidl et al,[15] 2008	Real-time telemedicine for high-priority communication Store and forward since medication orders were transmitted to the telepharmacist via order scanning technology	Asynchronous and synchronous	Responsive to request for requested consultation Responsive to problems identified during medication order review	Telephone, telemedicine note-writing system, video conferencing	After-hours care and expanded daylight services to smaller hospitals. Review of pharmacy orders, order verification, consultation with the nurse and physicians for medication preparation, compatibility, and administration

(continued on next page)

Table 2
(continued)

Reference	Type of Telepharmacy	Type of Communication	Model of Care	Mode of Communication	Pharmacy Service Provided
Forni et al,[13] 2010	Real-time telemedicine Store and forward since a custom sedation tool extracted information from the ICU electronic medical record	Asynchronous and synchronous	Responsive to problems identified during medication order review	Telephone, electronic task list, e-mail	After-hours care and supplement to daylight activities by critical care pharmacist. Services provided were medication order review, drug information, pharmacotherapy and pharmacokinetic consultation, systematic medication and allergy reconciliation. Real-time interventions on sedation protocol noncompliance
Keeys et al,[18] 2014	Real-time telemedicine for high-priority communication Store and forward since medication lists were transmitted to the telepharmacist	Asynchronous and synchronous	Responsive because interaction occurred if a discrepancy was identified	Telephone, facsimile, or in-house e-mail	Review of medication orders by a pharmacist at hospital discharge for after hours and to supplement the activities of the daylight pharmacist. Service was originally piloted for critical care patients

| Amkreutz et al,[14] 2018 | Real-time telemedicine for tele-ICU rounds Store and forward since medication data are uploaded to electronic medical record and used later during telerounds | Synchronous | Scheduled since all recommendations were provided during the interdisciplinary tele-ICU team rounds that included the on-site ICU staff | Videoconferencing | Telepharmacy consultations offered during the day on weekdays in conjunction with existing tele-ICU services. Medication safety check performed for drug-drug interactions, dosage adjustments, potentially inadequate medications for elderly patients |

same as with any telemedicine service, including cost (startup and maintenance), legal issues, confidentiality concerns, reimbursement, and licensing issues across state lines. Telepharmacy requires substantial forethought, including key stakeholder involvement with the planning, the development of service standards (especially if telepharmacy service is outsourced), consideration of the interplay with existing pharmacy services (if applicable), and outlining workflows, a priori. Also, reimbursement for telepharmacy services is not delineated at this time.

There is clearly a cost for technology such as hardware, software, and communication strategies between locations. Although several of these costs are upfront costs, there are still continuous costs for maintenance, upgrades, and security. There is a cost for the pharmacy and information technology personnel. Depending on how many sites the central telepharmacy services, the costs could be dispersed over the sites, thus alleviating some of the burden. The question arises in understanding whether there is a return on the investment. Cost saving for telepharmacy services provided in the ICU was $121,966 for 817 pharmacist interventions or $1340 per day.[15] This saving is approximately $175 per intervention in 2018 dollars. Another study conducted outside of the ICU provided an estimated average cost per intervention of $115 in present-day value.[22] It therefore seems that approximately $150 per intervention is a reasonable estimate.

The regulations for providing telepharmacy services are highly variable by state. For example, Medicaid reimburses for provider-delivered services for pharmacologic management on an individual-recipient basis but excludes pharmacy services as reimbursable. California law states, "remote dispensing site pharmacies are permitted to dispense or provide pharmaceutical care services in medically underserved areas."[23] Many laws are focused on drug dispensing and not pharmacologic management. Also, many state boards of pharmacy have developed their own interpretations of telepharmacy, so it is essential to find the laws that are applicable to the state in which the clinician practices. Even less clear is the provision of telepharmacy services across state lines. **Box 1**[23-26] provides a list of useful Web sites with state regulations for telemedicine services. Newer telemedicine laws, as in the state of New Jersey, are offering a broader definition of health care providers, supporting provision by a variety of different providers.

TELESTROKE

Based on the morbidity and mortality associated with stroke, the timing of potentially lifesaving and neuroprotective interventions, and the lack of expertise and resources

Box 1	
Reference Web sites for regulations by state	
Organization or Name of Document	**URL**
American Medical Association[23]	https://www.ama-assn.org/system/files/2018-10/ama-chart-telemedicine-patient-physician-relationship.pdf
Center for Connected Health Policy[24]	https://www.cchpca.org/telehealth-policy/current-state-laws-and-reimbursement-policies?jurisdiction=72&category=All&topic=All
National Association of Boards of Pharmacy[25]	https://nabp.pharmacy/wp-content/uploads/2016/07/Innovations_June_July_Final.pdf
Telepharmacy Rules and Statutes: A 50-state Survey[26]	https://www.public-health.uiowa.edu/rupri/publications/other/Telepharmacy%20Rules%20Article.pdf

to meet the demand for caring of patients with stroke, telestroke is the most rapidly evolving application of telemedicine in health care in the United States at both prehospital and hospital levels. Clinical studies have shown the efficacy of telestroke in stroke recognition, image interpretation, increase in intravenous (IV) administration of tissue plasminogen activator (tPA), and recognition of patients' suitability for endovascular interventions.[27–34]

Multiple studies have evaluated the effect of telemedicine networks on stroke care.[35] Recently, the concept of mobile stroke units linked to telemedicine networks for stroke care was assessed in a feasibility study.[30] Using the RP-Express (InTouch Health Inc., Santa Barbara, CA) over fourth-generation (4G) broadband cellular network technology and Long-term Evolution (LTE) networks, simulated evaluations of patients with stroke at the prehospital level (Prehospital Utility of Rapid Stroke evaluation Using In-ambulance Telemedicine [PURSUIT] study) were deemed feasible and accurate. Prehospital mobile stroke unit assessments led to increased rates of IV tPA administration and reduced the time to IV tPA administration compared with regular ambulance transports to emergency departments (EDs).[36–38]

In the ED, the efficiency and accuracy of recognition of stroke syndromes were shown by the National Institutes of Health (NIH)–funded Stroke Team Remote Evaluation using a Digital Observation Camera study (Stroke-DOC).[27] Two-way audiovisual consultation was superior to telephone-based consultation in accurately identifying patients with stroke, yielding a higher rate of IV tPA administration with a similar incidence in intracerebral hemorrhage, but without effect on overall functional outcome.[27]

In addition, other studies have shown that emergency interpretation of electronically transferred images (computed tomography scans) during telestroke care is both feasible and accurate.[39] In the new era of recanalization for stroke with large-vessel occlusion,[40] telestroke has assisted in improving recognition of patients with stroke in need of endovascular therapies, leading to better functional outcomes and quality of life.[32–34,41]

Telestroke networks assist in the delivery of stroke care to patients with ischemic stroke. Improvements in triage, recognition, and access to lifesaving interventions are supported by robust evidence. Moreover, it seems that there is no difference in outcomes for patients treated directly at comprehensive stroke centers compared with patients transferred from remote hospitals.[42] The benefits may extend beyond patients with ischemic stroke. Because early recognition of intracranial hemorrhages is fundamental for the exclusion of IV thrombolytic administration, telemedicine evaluation provides a unique way to identify this and other conditions that may mimic an ischemic stroke. In addition, other potentially life-threatening neurologic injuries that need expert neurocritical or neurosurgical interventions can be identified with this technology.[43,44] Inherent risks of telemedicine technology use are potential loss of patient confidentiality.

Consistent with the descriptions proposed by the ATA, the type of communication necessary for telestroke is real time, synchronous, and responsive based on the urgency of the communication.[4–8] Also, the ATA provides guidelines for the implementation of telestroke models. The ATA describes 2 different operational models: distributive and hub-spoke. In the distributive model, an independent agency or corporation or affiliated group of telestroke physicians provides services to different participating sites. In the hub-spoke model, a comprehensive stroke center or academic facility provides expert remote telestroke services to participating or affiliated spoke sites.[45] Regardless of the model, telestroke service providers should implement the appropriate operational structure to satisfy the ATA standards (Box 2).

Box 2
Key points from American Telemedicine Association administrative guidelines for telestroke services

- Organization
  - Agreement for standard operating procedures
  - Administrative policies/procedures based on relevant government agencies
- Leadership
  - Identification of executive leadership (Stroke Champions)
  - Implementation of procedures to track patient safety and quality
- Roles and responsibilities
  - Specific roles of stakeholders (eg, administrators, information technology personnel, human resources, legal, finance, medical providers)
  - Identification of site physician director, program manager, stroke champion, and so forth
- Human resources management
  - To support orientation, staff development, and competency of telestroke program
  - Development of guidelines for processes within the telestroke network (eg, emergency medical services, emergency department, intensive care unit, stroke unit, Rehab)
- Accreditation/certification/regulatory
  - Providers must maintain current certification and/or state licensure
  - Maintenance of liability insurance
- Privacy and confidentiality
  - Incorporation of Health Insurance Portability and Accountability Act compliant systems
- Fiscal management
  - Establishment of budgets
  - Definition of investments costs and compensation
- Patient records and documentation
  - Define processes and policies for documentation and maintenance of medical records
- Work flow and communication
  - Develop policies for adequate patient sign out and handoff
- Training
  - Develop adequate training for providers in key areas related to operation of telestroke network: information technology, electronic medical record, picture archiving and communication system, patient assessment with National Institute for Health Stroke Scale
- Quality outcomes
  - Establishment of benchmarks tracking quality and performance
  - Quality indicators for administration, information technology, and clinical components
- Patient rights
  - Develop strategies to keep patients and families informed about the role and objectives of telestroke networks

Data from Demaerschalk BM, Berg J, Chong BW, et al. American Telemedicine Association: telestroke guidelines. Telemed J E Health 2017;23:376–89.

The basic requirement for telestroke evaluations is a secure and reliable communication link with the high-definition audiovisual interface. Ideally, the platform and network should be rapidly responsive, and with 24/7/365 on-call technology support for troubleshooting. Commercially available platforms rely on fast broadband connections for adequate telemedicine evaluations. Although broadband connections provide undisputed reliability, wireless (3G, 4G, LTE, and Wi-Fi)-based communications have been implemented to extend the range and access of telemedicine platforms. The use of telemedicine services over Wi-Fi has already been tested and found

Reference	Type of Teledialysis	Type of Communication	Model of Care	Mode of Communication	Service Provided
Montanari et al,[52] 1992 Rumpsfeld et al,[53] 2005	Remote patient monitoring	Asynchronous and synchronous are possible	Responsive	Telephone or video communication is likely	Remote, central guidance of hemodialysis provided in a rural site

Table 3
Description of teledialysis services for acute care

feasible.[43,46–48] In the United States, the Health Insurance Portability and Accountability Act (HIPAA) requires any communication disclosing the patients' personal and health information to be secured with encrypted transmissions to protect the patients' confidentiality. Similarly, telemedicine evaluations are now part of electronic medical records providing substantial support for time-sensitive interventions. All centers must recognize the need to protect information and the importance of adhering to those standards.

TELEDIALYSIS

Teledialysis used for the management of patients receiving care in their homes seems common; however, the use of teledialysis for acute care is less clear. Similar to the idea of expanding services for other subsets of telemedicine, teledialysis may be a viable option. Jhaveri and colleagues.[49] performed a systematic review to analyze the outcomes of teledialysis involving supervision to deliver active treatment to rural patients. Only 3 studies were identified that met these criteria. Overall, patient satisfaction was positive and afforded the patients additional independent living.[50,51] The data describing remote oversight of dialysis delivered in a rural hospital for acute care are scant (**Table 3**).[52,53] A survey conducted in Canadian hospitals indicates that about 50% of respondents (36 of 73 hospitals) use continuous renal replacement therapy (CRRT), but CRRT is recommended in the 2012 Kidney Disease: Improving Global Outcomes (KDIGO) guidelines for hemodynamically unstable patients.[54,55] Future application of teledialysis for critically ill patients could be in resource-limited or expertise-limited institutions trying to adopt CRRT. Although teledialysis service for acute care seems possible as a means of efficiently providing qualified patient care to a setting in need, more information is needed to ascertain the value. There are insufficient data and outcome assessments to offer definitive conclusions for benefit and risks. Legal considerations specific to teledialysis have not been outlined. Because teledialysis is a subset of telemedicine, it would be prudent to follow the existing regulations. The pilot test of remote teledialysis services for acute care indicated a financial loss of about $35,000 in present-day value,[53] although the economic implications for teledialysis of critically ill patients is still unknown. Clinicians are just beginning to delve into the use of teledialysis for acute care, and more research is required to fully elucidate appropriate applications and related patient outcomes.

TELE–EMERGENCY MEDICINE

Tele–emergency medicine is a means of providing consultation between a central ED and a rural ED for real-time, synchronous communication typically involving video conferencing. Over 2.5 years of evaluation of 21 hospitals, only 3.5% of encounters used the tele-emergency services and most commonly for circulatory compromises, injury, mental and respiratory compromises, and symptomatic control.[56] Among patients with toxicologic emergencies for which expertise in management at the hospital may be lacking, tele-emergency and telepharmacy services may be suitable options.[57] Tele–emergency services with overt critical care implications are real-time, synchronous audio and video communication between emergency physicians and emergency medical services for prehospital evaluation of seriously injured patients with trauma.[58]

The benefits to tele–emergency services are improving clinical quality, expanding the patient care team, and providing focused patient-centered encounters that are aligned with other telehealth services.[59] In addition, unnecessary transfers from a rural hospital are avoided, resulting in a cost avoidance of $3823 per transfer avoided.[60] Also, tele–emergency services have aided in shortening the time to care and improving the recruitment of family physicians.[59]

OTHER TELEHEALTH SERVICES

Telehealth is provided for a variety of other services, such as tele–transition of care, teledermatology, teleprocedures, telerehabilitation, teleophthalmology, and teleoncology. It seems that these services have not reached and/or are not applicable to critical care. As more telehealth services reach the care of critically ill patients, it will be essential to describe services and outcomes for general adoption.

SUMMARY

As more specialized care gets centralized in centers of excellence, patients transported to community and rural hospitals may be at a disadvantage at the time of accessing expertise or receiving advanced care. In this setting, telemedicine models provide a justification to equalize care across different levels. There is still a lack of empirical research, including best practices and resultant outcomes for telemedicine models, but, if proved to be beneficial, this technology has the potential to equalize geographic discrepancies in the distribution of specialized care. With the overwhelming expansion of telemedicine services to subsets of acute care, addressing limitations related to regulations, confidentiality, reimbursement, and licensure should be a priority.

REFERENCES

1. Adler-Milstein J, Kvedar J, Bates DW. Telehealth among US hospitals: several factors, including state reimbursement and licensure policies, influence adoption. Health Aff (Millwood) 2014;33:207–15.

2. Williams AM, Bhatti UF, Alam HS, et al. The role of telemedicine in postoperative care. Mhealth 2018;4:11.

3. Monegain B. Telemedicine to soar past $30B 2015. Available at: https://www.healthcareitnews.com/news/telemedicine-poised-grow-big-time. Accessed October 21, 2018.

4. American Telemedicine Association. Telemedicine glossary. Available at: http://thesource.americantelemed.org/resources/telemedicine-glossary. Accessed October 21, 2018.

5. Davis TM, Barden C, Dean S, et al. American telemedicine association guidelines for teleICU operations. Telemed J E Health 2016;22:971–80.

6. Telligen Health Information Technology Center. Telehealth start-up and resource guide 2014. Available at: https://www.healthit.gov/sites/default/files/playbook/pdf/telehealth-startup-and-resource-guide.pdf. Accessed October 21, 2018.

7. Center for Medicare and Medicaid Services. Telemedicine. Available at: https://www.medicaid.gov/medicaid/benefits/telemed/index.html. Accessed October 21, 2018.

8. eVisit. The ultimate telemedicine guide. What is telemedicine? 2018. Available at: https://evisit.com/resources/what-is-telemedicine/. Accessed October 21, 2018.

9. Khunlertkit A, Carayon P. Contributions of tele-intensive care unit (Tele-ICU) technology to quality of care and patient safety. J Crit Care 2013;28:315.e1-12.

10. Alexander E, Bulter CD, Darr A, et al. ASHP statement on telepharmacy. Am J Health Syst Pharm 2017;74:e236–41.

11. Poudel A, Nissen LM. Telepharmacy: a pharmacist's perspective on the clinical benefits and challenges. Integr Pharm Res Pract 2016;26:75–82.

12. Niznik JD, He H, Kane-Gill SL. Impact of clinical pharmacist services delivered via telemedicine in the outpatient for ambulatory care setting: a systematic review. Res Social Adm Pharm 2018;14:707–17.

13. Forni A, Skehan N, Harman CA, et al. Evaluation of the impact of a tele-ICU pharmacists on the management of sedation in the critically ill mechanically ventilated patients. Ann Pharmacother 2010;44:432–8.

14. Amkreutz J, Lenssen R, Marz G, et al. Medication safety in a German telemedicine centre: implementation of a telepharmaceutical expert consultation in addition to existing tele-intensive care unit services. J Telemed Telecare 2018. https://doi.org/10.1177/1357633X18799796.

15. Meidl TM, Woller TW, Iglar AM, et al. Implementation of pharmacy services in a telemedicine intensive care unit. Am J Health Syst Pharm 2008;65:1464–9.

16. Strnad K, Shoulders BR, Smithburger PL, et al. A systematic review of ICU and non-ICU clinical pharmacy services using telepharmacy. Ann Pharmacother 2018;52:1250–8.

17. Keeys CA, Dandurand K, Harris J, et al. Providing nighttime pharmaceutical services through telepharmacy. Am J Health Syst Pharm 2002;59:716–21.

18. Keeys C, Kalejaiye B, Skinner M, et al. Pharmacist-managed inpatient discharge medication reconciliation: a combined onsite and telepharmacy model. Am J Health Syst Pharm 2014;71:2159–66.

19. Kane SL, Weber RJ, Dasta JF. The impact of critical care pharmacists on enhancing patient outcomes. Intensive Care Med 2003;29:691–8.

20. Bauer SR, Kane-Gill SL. Outcome assessment of critical care pharmacist services. Hosp Pharm 2016;51:507–13.

21. Leape LL, Cullen DJ, Clapp MD, et al. Pharmacist participation on physicians rounds and adverse drug events in the intensive care unit. JAMA 1999;21(283):267–70.

22. Garrelts JC, Gagnon M, Eisenberg C, et al. Impact of telepharmacy in a multihospital health system. Am J Health Syst Pharm 2010;67:1456–62.

23. Center for Connected Health Policy. Current state laws & reimbursement policies 2018. Available at: https://www.cchpca.org/telehealth-policy/current-state-laws-and-reimbursement-policies?jurisdiction=72&category=All&topic=All. Accessed October 21, 2018.

24. American Medical Association. 50-state survey: establishment of a patient-physician relationship via telemedicine. Available at: https://www.ama-assn.org/sites/default/files/media-browser/specialty%20group/arc/ama-chart-telemedicine-patient-physician-relationship.pdf. Accessed Oct. 21, 2018.

25. National Association of Boards of Pharmacy. Telepharmacy: the new frontier of patient care and professional practice 2017. Available at: https://nabp. pharmacy/wp-content/uploads/2016/07/Innovations_June_July_Final.pdf. Accessed October 21, 2018.

26. Tzanetakos G, Ullrich F, Mueller K. Telepharmacy rules and statutes: a 50-state survey. Rural Policy Brief 2017;4:1–4.

27. Meyer BC, Raman R, Hemmen T, et al. Efficacy of site-independent telemedicine in the STRokE DOC trial: a randomised, blinded, prospective study. Lancet Neurol 2008;7:787–95.

28. Agrawal K, Raman R, Ernstrom K, et al. Accuracy of stroke diagnosis in telestroke-guided tissue plasminogen activator patients. J Stroke Cerebrovasc Dis 2016;25:2942–6.

29. Chalouhi N, Dressler JA, Kunkel ES, et al. Intravenous tissue plasminogen activator administration in community hospitals facilitated by telestroke service. Neurosurgery 2013;73:667–71 [discussion: 71–2].

30. Van Hooff RJ, Cambron M, Van Dyck R, et al. Prehospital unassisted assessment of stroke severity using telemedicine: a feasibility study. Stroke 2013;44:2907–9.

31. Mitchell JR, Sharma P, Modi J, et al. A smartphone client-server teleradiology system for primary diagnosis of acute stroke. J Med Internet Res 2011;13:e31.

32. Pedragosa A, Alvarez-Sabin J, Rubiera M, et al. Impact of telemedicine on acute management of stroke patients undergoing endovascular procedures. Cerebrovasc Dis 2012;34:436–42.

33. Barlinn J, Gerber J, Barlinn K, et al. Acute endovascular treatment delivery to ischemic stroke patients transferred within a telestroke network: a retrospective observational study. Int J Stroke 2017;12:502–9.

34. Kepplinger J, Dzialowski I, Barlinn K, et al. Emergency transfer of acute stroke patients within the East Saxony telemedicine stroke network: a descriptive analysis. Int J Stroke 2014;9:160–5.

35. Muller-Barna P, Hubert GJ, Boy S, et al. TeleStroke units serving as a model of care in rural areas: 10-year experience of the TeleMedical project for integrative stroke care. Stroke 2014;45:2739–44.

36. Gyrd-Hansen D, Olsen KR, Bollweg K, et al. Cost-effectiveness estimate of prehospital thrombolysis: results of the PHANTOM-S study. Neurology 2015;84: 1090–7.

37. Ebinger M, Kunz A, Wendt M, et al. Effects of golden hour thrombolysis: a prehospital acute neurological treatment and optimization of medical care in stroke (PHANTOM-S) substudy. JAMA Neurol 2015;72:25–30.

38. Kunz A, Ebinger M, Geisler F, et al. Functional outcomes of pre-hospital thrombolysis in a mobile stroke treatment unit compared with conventional care: an observational registry study. Lancet Neurol 2016;15:1035–43.

39. Pexman JH, Barber PA, Hill MD, et al. Use of the Alberta Stroke Program Early CT Score (ASPECTS) for assessing CT scans in patients with acute stroke. AJNR Am J Neuroradiol 2001;22:1534–42.

40. Goyal M, Menon BK, van Zwam WH, et al. Endovascular thrombectomy after large-vessel ischaemic stroke: a meta-analysis of individual patient data from five randomised trials. Lancet 2016;387:1723–31.

41. McAdams M, Murphy J, DePrince M, et al. Assessing the impact of care in a telemedicine-based stroke network using patient-centered health-related quality-of-life outcomes. Eur Stroke J 2016;1:121.

42. Wechsler LR, Demaerschalk BM, Schwamm LH, et al. Telemedicine quality and outcomes in stroke: a scientific statement for healthcare professionals from the American Heart Association/American Stroke Association. Stroke 2017;48:e3–25.
43. Vespa PM, Miller C, Hu X, et al. Intensive care unit robotic telepresence facilitates rapid physician response to unstable patients and decreased cost in neurointensive care. Surg Neurol 2007;67:331–7.
44. Vespa P. Robotic telepresence in the intensive care unit. Crit Care 2005;9:319–20.
45. Demaerschalk BM, Berg J, Chong BW, et al. American Telemedicine Association: telestroke guidelines. Telemed J E Health 2017;23:376–89.
46. Craig J, Patterson V, Russell C, et al. Interactive videoconsultation is a feasible method for neurological in-patient assessment. Eur J Neurol 2000;7:699–702.
47. Khan K, Shuaib A, Whittaker T, et al. Telestroke in northern Alberta: a two year experience with remote hospitals. Can J Neurol Sci 2010;37:808–13.
48. Rincon F, Vibbert M, Childs V, et al. Implementation of a model of robotic telepresence (RTP) in the neuro-ICU: effect on critical care nursing team satisfaction. Neurocrit Care 2012;17:97–101.
49. Jhaveri D, Larkins S, Sabesan S. Telestroke, tele-oncology and teledialysis: a systematic review to analyse the outcomes of active therapies delivered with telemedicine support. J Telemed Telecare 2015;21:181–8.
50. Rygh E, Arild E, Johnsen E, et al. Choosing to live with home dialysis-patients' experiences and potential for telemedicine support: a qualitative study. BMC Nephrol 2012;13:13.
51. Whitten P, Buis L. Use of telemedicine for haemodialysis: perceptions of patients and health-care providers, and clinical effects. J Telemed Telecare 2008;14:75–8.
52. Montanari A, Briganti M, Emiliani G, et al. Can teledialysis help in the clinical management of patients on remote hemodialysis? Int J Artif Organs 1992;15:397–400.
53. Rumpsfeld M, Arild E, Norum J, et al. Telemedicine in haemodialysis: a university department and two remote satellites linked together as one common workplace. J Telemed Telecare 2005;11:251–5.
54. Bourbounnais FF, Sivar S, Tucker SM. Continuous renal replacement therapy practices in Canadian hospitals: where are we now? Can J Crit Care Nurs 2016;27:17–22.
55. Kellum JA, Lameire N, KDIGO AKI guideline work group. Diagnosis, evaluation, and management of acute kidney injury: a KDIGO summary (Part 1). Crit Care 2013;17:205.
56. Ward MM, Ulrich E, MacKinney AC, et al. Tele-emergency utilization: in what clinical situations is tele-emergency activated? J Telemed Telecare 2016;22:25–31.
57. Russi CS, Mattson AE, Smars PA, et al. Ethylene glycol and methanol ingestion care for by tele-emergency pharmacy and tele-emergency medicine. J Telemed Telecare 2018. https://doi.org/10.1177/1357633X18778631.
58. Eder PA, Reime B, Wurmb T. Prehospital telemedical emergency management of severely injured trauma patients. Methods Inf Med 2018. https://doi.org/10.3414/ME18-05-0001.
59. Mueller KJ, Potter AJ, MacKinney AC, et al. Lessons from tele-emergency: improving care quality and health outcomes by expanding support for rural care systems. Health Aff (Millwood) 2014;33:228–34.
60. Natafgi N, Shane DM, Ullrich F, et al. Using tele-emergency to avoid patient transfers in rural emergency departments: an assessment of costs of benefits. J Telemed Telecare 2018;24:193–201.

Moving?

Make sure your subscription moves with you!

To notify us of your new address, find your **Clinics Account Number** (located on your mailing label above your name), and contact customer service at:

Email: journalscustomerservice-usa@elsevier.com

800-654-2452 (subscribers in the U.S. & Canada)
314-447-8871 (subscribers outside of the U.S. & Canada)

Fax number: 314-447-8029

Elsevier Health Sciences Division
Subscription Customer Service
3251 Riverport Lane
Maryland Heights, MO 63043

*To ensure uninterrupted delivery of your subscription, please notify us at least 4 weeks in advance of move.

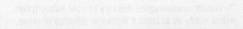

Printed and bound by CPI Group (UK) Ltd, Croydon, CR0 4YY

03/10/2024

01040480-0012